MEANING & MEDICINE

MEANING & MEDICINE

Lessons from a Doctor's Tales of Breakthrough and Healing

LARRY DOSSEY, M.D.

BANTAM BOOKS

NEW YORK · TORONTO · LONDON · SYDNEY · AUCKLAND

Many of the clinical cases in this book are based on actual events occurring in the author's practice of internal medicine. All names have been changed to preserve confidentiality.

MEANING & MEDICINE

A BANTAM BOOK

Publishing History
Bantam hardcover edition published December 1991
Bantam trade paperback edition / December 1992

See page 289 for credits.

Book design by Jaya Dayal.

Library of Congress Catalog Card Number 91-3598.

ISBN 0-553-37081-2

PUBLISHED SIMULTANEOUSLY IN THE UNITED STATES AND CANADA

Bantam Books are published by Bantam Books, a division of Bantam Doubleday Dell Publishing Group, Inc. Its trademark, consisting of the words "Bantam Books" and the portrayal of a rooster, is Registered in U.S. Patent and Trademark Office and in other countries. Marca Registrada. Bantam Books, 666 Fifth Avenue, New York, New York 10103.

PRINTED IN THE UNITED STATES OF AMERICA

RRH   0 9 8 7 6 5 4 3 2 1

For
PROFESSOR D. S. KOTHARI

Meaning is being.

—DAVID BOHM

Acknowledgments

Although I owe thanks to more people than I can name for helping shape the concepts that follow, I want especially to acknowledge Professor D. S. Kothari, to whom this book is dedicated. Dr. Kothari, a physicist, worked at the legendary Cavendish laboratory at Cambridge University and the Niels Bohr Institute. A pioneer in applying nuclear and quantum principles to the theory of white dwarf stars, he is perhaps India's best-known living scientist. He is professor emeritus at the University of Delhi and chancellor of Jawaharlal Nehru University in Delhi. As chairman of the University Grants Commission of India from 1961 to 1973, he guided the development of science throughout all of India, the world's largest democracy. Dr. Kothari had come across my book *Space, Time & Medicine,*[1] which occasioned the beginning of a stimulating correspondence. An unforgettable experience for me was receiving his landmark paper "Atom and Self." Published in an Indian scientific journal in 1980, it is one of the most profound discussions of the mind-body problem I have ever discovered.[2] It was my great honor to meet Professor Kothari when I was invited in January 1988 to deliver the annual Mahatma Gandhi Memorial Lecture at the Gandhi Peace Foundation in New Delhi. Dr. Kothari spoke the languages of modern physics and the ancient Upanishads with equal profundity and grace. In his life and philosophy he has honored the realities of the physical, mental, and spiritual as few scientists I have known. Our conversations and the communication that has followed have for me been memorable and inspiring, and have contributed in no small measure to the ideas set forth in this volume.

To Leslie Meredith, executive editor at Bantam, I owe special appreciation. With her insight and gentle patience, she has been a beacon throughout this writing, helping me keep my goal in sight.

I wish also to thank an unheralded class of healers who have been my continual teachers, who have taught me lessons I never learned in medical school: nurses. For generations, the profession of nursing has given safe harbor to many of the entities made homeless by an impersonal science, including love, caring, and meaning in healing. Anything I understand about the function of meaning in health and illness I owe largely to them—especially one particular nurse, from whom I've learned most: Barbara, my colleague and wife.

To Juan and Rosa Ortega, special thanks for two decades of lessons in meaning under sun, stars, and storms, and around campfires on mountaintops and deserts.

Finally, to the patients who have shared their stories, I extend my gratitude and love.

Contents

Talking Out the Worms

> Everything in this world has a hidden meaning. . . .
> Men, animals, trees, stars, they are all hierogly-
> phics. . . . When you see them, you do not under-
> stand them. You think they are really men, animals,
> trees, stars. It is only years later . . . that you
> understand. . . .
>
> —NIKOS KAZANTZAKIS
> *Zorba the Greek*[1]

I first began to think about the meaning of illness when I was five
years old, growing up on a small sharecropper cotton farm in central
Texas. In the 1940s, life on those bleak blackland prairies was an
endless round of bank foreclosures, boll weevils, and drought. As an
additional nuisance, during the summertime the few head of cattle
small cotton farmers owned were in constant danger of attack by
screwworms, *cochliomyia hominivorax,* a devilish pest that was particularly well named. Female flies would lay their eggs in any open
wound of an animal and small white maggots would hatch. These
would bore like screws through the animal's tissues, tearing away
the flesh and leaving gigantic holes in their wake. As a consequence
the animal could be maimed for life or, not uncommonly, die of the
accompanying infection.

Like physicians making rounds, farmers continually surveyed
their cattle during the summer, looking for any cut or wound that had

become infected. Treatment was gruesome. The animal had to be captured and immobilized while the squirming mass of maggots was scraped from the infected site. Then as the animal writhed in pain, the blood-raw cavity was doused with a concoction of foul-smelling chemicals to cauterize it and destroy any remaining screwworms and unhatched eggs. But sometimes the treatment didn't work.

One day, after multiple attempts, my father gave up on treating a young calf with a gaping wound on its flank. It could not walk, was in constant agony, would not eat, and was slowly dying. Looking at the calf, my father simply said, "Let's go get Maria."

I had never heard of Maria and had no idea what my father had in mind. We drove for miles down a narrow unpaved road into the prairie countryside, eventually turning onto a lane that led to a small, run-down shack situated conspicuously in the middle of a small cotton field. Maria and her family lived here; they were Mexicans who subsisted as farm laborers. After a lengthy conversation in Spanish, which I couldn't understand, she followed my father back to the car and returned with us to our farm and the dying calf, saying nothing the entire trip.

Maria, I later discovered, was a *curandera,* a folk healer. The local farmers kept her in reserve for the really tough cases. They frequently preferred her to the expensive local veterinarian who, in those days before antibiotics, was often as helpless as they against overwhelming screwworm infections.

Maria got out of the car without a word and began walking to the barnyard where the sick calf lay.

"What's she going to do?" I whispered to my father.

"She's going to talk out the worms," he said.

I was completely confused by his reply, stunned to think that worms could actually converse with humans. I tried to coax an explanation from my father, by nature a reticent man, but could not. I began to trail after Maria, not wanting to miss anything, but my father, towering above me, placed his hand on my shoulder and said, "Son, we can't watch her. She has to be alone."

Disappointed, I viewed Maria from a considerable distance. I saw her dark figure kneel before the calf, which was on its side. It seemed curiously unafraid of her. She made several passes with her hands over the animal and then, after she remained still for many minutes, her lips began to move.

After a half hour the ritual ended, and this mysterious woman signaled to my father that she was finished by raising her head slowly and fixing her gaze on him. He nodded to me that it was okay, and we both walked to the barnyard. Curiously, my father paid almost no attention to the calf; he seemed to have no doubts whatsoever about the results of her "therapy." Maria walked with us to the car, and we retraced our route over the country roads on the long drive back to her house. My father escorted her to the front porch of the shack, where they began to converse. After several minutes he paid Maria a small sum and we left once more to return home.

"What did she say to you, Dad?"

"Maria knows why the calf is sick. She says it has a strong will and is always misbehaving. It got the cut on its flank from barbed wire when it tried to escape the pasture and the rest of the cows. She says the infection is the price it has paid, but that it is a very smart calf and has learned its lesson. She made a bargain with the worms. She told them they have succeeded in teaching the calf a valuable lesson. But if they stay, the calf will die and they will eventually die with it. It would be better for everyone if they leave now and spare the calf."

"But what if they don't?"

"She threatened them with stronger measures if they stay. She says the worms listened and are afraid. They are leaving now and the calf is going to be all right."

"But how does Maria *know* all this?" My father, sensing my pained confusion, looked at me and smiled.

"Maria," he said patiently, "knows what things *mean*."

It was late when we arrived home, and while Dad finished the chores in the moonlight, I grabbed a flashlight and ran to the barnyard and the calf. I had to have a look for myself. The calf was standing, for the first time in days, eating from a trough. There were no worms in sight in the gaping wound, which—did I imagine it?—was smaller. In a few days it had healed completely and the calf was fine.

The Knave of Hearts: "I don't believe there's an atom
of meaning in it."

The King: "If there's no meaning in it, that saves a
world of trouble, you know, as we needn't try to
find any. [But] I seem to see some meaning . . .
after all."

—LEWIS CARROLL
Alice in Wonderland

I soon forgot about screwworms because they ceased to be much of
a problem. An effective eradication program for them was developed,
based on releasing sterile male flies into the environment. They mated
with the females, and the resulting eggs, deposited by females into
open wounds, were infertile and did not hatch.

I forgot, that is, until twenty-five years later when I was finishing
my residency in internal medicine.

As the admissions officer of the day at a very large teaching
hospital, it was my duty to screen all applicants who wished to be
admitted to the Internal Medicine Service. It was great training
because, with the enormous volume of patients, one would eventually see almost every conceivable illness, even exotic ones like—as it
turned out—screwworms.

Jack, a patient seeking medical care, was a farm worker who
drifted from job to job. He loved farm life and had once owned a
small plot in east Texas. However, "bad luck" and a severe drinking
problem resulted in the forfeiture of his land and his current status as
a wandering laborer. Jack was a maverick at heart. He had always
seen himself as not fitting in—not because of any shortcoming on his
part, as he saw it, but because "the system" was always stacked
against him.

"Why do you want to see a doctor?" I asked.

"I have screwworms, Doc," he replied. Jack was obviously
embarrassed.

It was a first for me. Never had I seen a human with this
affliction. I was sure he must be joking, but decided to play along.

"Show me."

Jack stood, turned, and removed his shirt, revealing a dirty
bandage at the junction of the back of his neck and right shoulder. I
began to remove it.

"Easy, Doc," he cautioned, obviously in pain.

I could not believe my eyes. Not since childhood had I seen maggots in living tissue, but here were several larvae, no mistaking it.

"How did this happen?"

Jack unfolded the tale in his slow drawl. He had been employed on a huge farm driving a tractor. One morning while plowing in a remote field he began to drink, thinking he would not be detected. By noon he was drunk and couldn't plow straight. He stopped the tractor at the end of the row and lay down in the shade of a large hackberry tree. Continuing to drink, he eventually passed out. As was his habit, Jack was working without a shirt—which, he reasoned, provided a female fly the chance to deposit her eggs in an open abrasion he had neglected. In a few days a painful sore formed at the site. Then one day, to his astonishment, a worm emerged from beneath the skin.

Although Jack could have been treated as an outpatient, we admitted him so everyone could learn from this extremely unusual case. Cutaneous worm infections of this sort were described in the medical literature—a condition known as myiasis—but none of us had ever seen one.[2]

The Infectious Disease Service placed Jack on antibiotics, and the Surgery Service treated the wound and changed his dressing daily. Overnight he became a celebrity around the hospital. Jack loved the attention and never passed up the chance to tell his tale to the constant stream of medical students, interns, and residents.

His infection was the final evidence Jack needed that society, "the system," was working against him. Simple illnesses weren't enough; in its vengeance the world had uniquely scourged him—screwworms! This allowed Jack to enlarge "the system" to include nature, which had obviously pulled out all the stops in its plot to make his life miserable.

I presented Jack's case at the weekly clinical conference, where unusual and challenging cases were discussed. I did not mention his colorful history and why he got the infection—his drinking, his inability to fit in socially, his hard luck. By then I had learned that disease "meant" nothing. In every case it was simply a physical process obeying the blind, neutral laws of nature.

After Jack was discharged from the hospital, I suddenly realized that this case had not been about him at all. In our eyes, "Jack" had not existed. He was only a body with an interesting diagnosis, a body that could have belonged to anyone.

I couldn't get Jack out of my mind. Suddenly old memories returned, and I began to think about the case of screwworms I had seen as a five-year-old. I was surprised that the elements of the memory were still so vivid: the willful calf, Maria, even the smell of the worm-killing chemicals. Even though the diagnoses of our respective cases were the same, how different Maria's approach to her case had been! She had seen meaning everywhere; other doctors and I had seen it nowhere. For her, the case could be understood only through meaning; for us, meaning was an obstruction to reason, something that got in the way of clear-headed judgment. Relying on the meaning behind the infection, Maria used words on the worms, while we blasted them with antibiotics and surgery. For Maria, meaning set the healing force in motion; for us it was a contaminant that could bring healing to a halt.

Wrestling with these issues after Jack was discharged, one night I had a dream. In it, Jack was still in the hospital. In spite of the antibiotics and surgery he was not getting better. Like my father's calf he was in great pain, could not eat, and was gradually dying. There was only one thing to do.

I drove down the country road to Maria's house and explained the situation to her. Agreeing to take on Jack's case, she returned with me to the hospital. We went straight to his room. I explained to Jack that Maria was here to talk out his worms. He immediately understood and was eager to proceed. Knowing that Maria needed to work alone, I stepped from the room and closed the door.

I was met in the hall by a retinue of white-coated colleagues, including the hospital administrator. No one was smiling and objections began to fly.

"A disgrace! She has no credentials!"

"She doesn't have hospital privileges!"

"The hospital's liability insurance doesn't cover this sort of thing!"

"Witchcraft! What if the media finds out!"

One fiery intern finally had enough. He reached for the door of Jack's room, determined to put an end to Maria's "therapy."

"Don't go in there; she has to work alone," I said. "Don't worry; there are no side effects. If it works you can give credit to the antibiotics and the surgeons."

Menacing and angry, the young intern looked at me and demanded, "Just what do you *mean* by all this?"

"How can you possibly ask me about meaning? Have you forgotten what we've been taught? Don't you remember there is *no* meaning to any of this?"

Suddenly the door sprang open and there was Jack—fully dressed, smiling, suitcase in hand, no more bandages. He appeared transformed. The impulsive intern spoke once again.

"What happened to *you*?" he demanded of Jack. The question was accusative and unkind.

"Maria explained why I got the infection and why I wasn't getting any better," Jack said. "She taught me to think about 'the system' in a different way. Now I know what my problem *means*. That's why it healed."

"You're a fool!" the intern retorted. "Disease means nothing. We all know it. Meaning just gets in the way."

By this time the crowd of young doctors was becoming a mob. But Jack was perfectly composed. As he had done when I first met him, he slowly removed his shirt and turned to demonstrate the infected wound. Nothing remained of it, not even a scar. Then Jack buttoned his shirt, grabbed his bag, and turned to leave. Like the Red Sea parting, the astonished group of physicians allowed him passage.

I entered the room to collect Maria and return her to her shack in the cotton field. The group of doctors trailed behind me and filled the room. But it was completely empty. Maria had vanished. On the bed was a large, irregular scrap of paper with a bold "**M**" scrawled on it with her signature.

"**M**oney," said the hospital administrator.

"**M**alpractice," said the derisive intern.

"**M**endacity," said a skeptical student.

Maria's gift, her lesson in Meaning, was lost.

Ten years later, after entering the private practice of internal medicine, I went to the coronary care unit one winter evening to make final hospital rounds for the day. That morning I had admitted Frank, a fifty-five-year-old patient, with chest pain resembling a heart attack. Through the day his course had been uneventful—no more pain, nausea, or irregular heartbeats. In fact, the day was so uneventful that Frank quickly became bored after he was confined to bed and "hooked up." Surveying his room, he noted the patterns of his heartbeat as they flowed steadily across the cardiac monitor mounted on the wall slightly behind him. An inquisitive sort, Frank was fascinated by this visual display, and he maneuvered his bedside table in such a way that he could watch the monitor behind him in the table's built-in mirror.

"Let me show you something on the monitor, Doc," he said later, as I entered his room. The digital display registered a heartbeat of seventy-five per minute, which soon fell to seventy, sixty-five, then sixty, where it remained. "Now watch this," Frank said. In a few moments the rate slowly crept up to eighty and stayed there. "I never knew I could do this before," he said, "but it's not hard if you concentrate."

Frank could see I was skeptical about his ability. I had known people could learn to control their heart rates through feedback techniques, but this usually required hours or days of practice, a sophisticated laboratory, and a skilled instructor. Frank was claiming to have discovered and mastered the technique on his own in only a few hours, despite the ominous atmosphere and constant interruptions of the coronary care unit and the grim possibility of having had a heart attack.

"You're not convinced, are you, Doc?" he said.

"No, Frank, I'm not," I responded honestly. On hearing this, he promptly performed the feat all over again. I felt Frank was taking pleasure in proving that "doctors don't know everything."

Each day Frank refined his skills and showed me every time I entered his room. He eventually was proved not to have had a heart attack, and on my final visit on his day of discharge I asked, "Frank, how do you do it? What do you concentrate on when you change your heart rate?" By this time, I was convinced that he truly had learned voluntary control, that the variations were not just the result of changes in breathing or of muscular contractions. Frank seemed obviously pleased that I'd finally taken the bait.

"It's simple," he replied. "I think about what my chest pains *mean* to me. If I let them mean a heart attack, I get anxious and the rate goes up. I see my heart damaged with the arteries clogged, I've lost my job, and I've got another heart attack on the way. But if I let the chest pain mean just a muscle ache or indigestion, I feel relieved and the heart rate comes down. Works like a charm!"

Frank's virtuoso performances were very impressive. Never before had I realized that a heart monitor could act as a "meaning meter." I wondered what other meaning meters surrounded us physicians and nurses—and our patients. Blood pressure cuffs? Stethoscopes? Thermometers?

I, and perhaps all modern physicians, have been trained to believe that Frank must be wrong. It is only the blind play of the atoms and molecules in the body that is important. These entities are unfeeling and unconscious, and their behavior is controlled by the neutral laws of nature. It is "bad science" to suggest that the perceived meanings of patients—in Frank's case, what he allowed his chest pain to mean to him—can affect the physical body. We believe that our *interpretation* of an event, the *significance* we attach to it, cannot possibly affect its course. For many, the physical is completely cut off from the mental, where meaning resides. That is why although stories like Frank's—as well as Maria's and Jack's—may be acknowledged as "interesting" or "amusing," they are largely ignored. Our culture believes these stories *must* be misleading and wrong, because they suggest the impossible: the action of mind on matter.

How could physicians have come to believe that the perceptions of our patients—their perceived meanings and significances, their thoughts, feelings, and emotions—do not matter? Every day we see "the mental" moving matter before our eyes. The will to live, for example, can forestall death by actually changing a host of physiological responses. In the placebo response, where a fake medication *means* the real drug to the patient, meaning moves matter dramatically. And, as every physician knows, heart attacks or sudden death can be brought on by emotional shock—by threatening, malevolent meanings, or even, as we shall see, positive, "good" meanings.

> [For archaic societies] *the world exists because it was*
> *created by the gods* . . . [thus] the existence of the
> world itself "means" something, "wants to say"
> something . . . the world is neither mute nor
> opaque . . . is not an inert thing without purpose
> or significance.
>
> —MIRCEA ELIADE[3]

The importance of meaning in our lives is reflected by the word's etymology. "Meaning" is derived from the Old English word *mænan,* "to recite, tell, intend, wish."[4] The word's origins suggest that without meaning our life is a blank page: we have no story to tell, nothing to recite. We have no content; we are a vacuous, empty shell. But meaning is connected also with intention and activity, as when we say we "mean" to do something. Without meaning, then, we have no intent in our life—no activity or energy, no goal to pursue. With no story to tell, no purpose, and no activity, we are as good as dead. This is not hyperbole. In fact, as many of the following stories show, physical death is literally the outcome of the various "no-meaning syndromes."

Not only can banishing meaning have a deadly effect on the body, it also has a deadening effect on the mind. Scientist-philosopher E. F. Schumacher noted:

> A person . . . entirely fixed in the philosophy of scientific
> materialistic Scientism, denying the reality of "invisibles" and
> confining his attention solely to what can be counted, mea-
> sured, and weighed, lives in a very poor world, so poor that
> he will experience it as a meaningless wasteland unfit for
> human habitation. Equally, if he sees it as nothing but an
> accidental collocation of atoms, he must needs agree with
> Bertrand Russell that the only rational attitude is one of
> "unyielding despair."[5]

Many observers have noted that scientific progress and the "information explosion" largely have failed to provide meaning in modern life. T. S. Eliot writes:

Where is the wisdom we have lost in knowledge?
Where is the knowledge we have lost in information?[6]

Archibald MacLeish says, "We are deluged with facts, but we have lost, or are losing, our human ability to *feel* them."[7]

Meaning makes the problems of life bearable, and without it we cannot process or integrate them. Yet, astonishingly, we have come to assume that *absence* of meaning is normal in modern life and we even sometimes attribute meaning to meaninglessness. This peculiar state of affairs is noted by psychiatrist Arthur J. Deikman:

> Existential despair is so culturally accepted that it is often defined as healthy. Consider the following extract from *The American Handbook of Psychiatry:*
>
>> To those who have obtained some wisdom in the process of reaching old age, death often assumes meaning as the proper outcome of life. It is nature's way of assuring much life and constant renewal. Time and customs change but the elderly tire of changing; it is time for others to take over, and the elderly person is willing to pass quietly from the scene.
>
> So we should end, according to the voice of reason, not with a bang or a whimper, but in a coma of increasing psychological fatigue.[8]

One of the most dismal pronouncements in this century on the nature of meaning comes from Sigmund Freud, the father of psychoanalysis, who felt that all values and meanings are nothing but defense mechanisms and reaction formations. Freud stated, "This alone I know with certainty, namely that men's value judgments are guided absolutely by their desire for happiness, and are therefore merely an attempt to bolster up their illusions by arguments."[9]

Meaning is the background against which we find answers to the great spiritual questions: Who am I? What is the purpose of my life—my true calling, my natural talent that I should exercise? Where did I come from, and where am I going? What are the limits of my freedom? Is there a God? If the great religions once provided the context of meaning in which answers to these questions could be found, it is no longer so; they appear to have lost much of their power and seem increasingly impotent and out-of-step in our complex world.

Once the fount of meaning, religion has come to blows with the modern scientific outlook and has been unable, by and large, to remain convincing. The religious and scientific perspectives are polarized over the question of meaning as perhaps no other. For religion, meaning is an intrinsic part of the world, part of the fabric of being behind all phenomena. For science, meaning does not exist. It is something we concoct, not something we discover in the world.

In addition to meaning, the concept of *mind* also has fared poorly at the hands of modern science. Mind experiences meaning. Mind is the faculty that—in the etymology of "meaning"—recites, intends, tells, or wishes. Without meaning, there is less need for mind; and without mind, there can be no meaning, as there is nothing for meaning to be meaningful *to*. It is not surprising, then, that mind and meaning have had similar fates.

One of the reasons medicine largely has denied mind and meaning as important factors in illness is the belief that it is "scientific" to do so. Physicians and medical researchers have experienced a genuine "physics envy" for over a century. This envy is not unique to medicine; other soft sciences—for example, education, economics, and psychology—have also wanted to embody the precision of physics. In medicine, following the lead of physics, we have striven to exclude subjectivity wherever it has arisen, which has meant denying a role for the mind and meaning in health and illness.

Perhaps it is time for physicians and medical researchers to reconsider the prohibition on meaning and "the mental" that is presumed to exist within physics. For Freeman Dyson, one of the preeminent physicists of our time, subatomic particles have mental properties. "Mind," he has said, "is already inherent in every electron."[10] Physicist David Bohm has proposed a similar possibility. "The question," he states, "is whether matter is rather crude and mechanical or whether it gets more and more subtle and becomes indistinguishable from what people have called mind."[11] For British physicist Paul Davies, the entire universe is not only conscious, it contains meaning as well. "The universe has organized its own self-awareness," he has said, "[which is] powerful evidence that there is 'something going on' behind it all. The impression of design is overwhelming . . . a meaning behind existence."[12]

These views are of course not shared by most physicists, and cannot be used as an absolute statement that a connection exists between the mental and the physical or that our minds affect our bodies. For this proof we must go to a domain about which physicists know almost nothing: the experiences of the Marias, Jacks, and Franks who have important tales to tell.

I have spent most of my life listening to people's stories. I've heard thousands of them—in examination rooms, hospital corridors, emergency departments, in parking lots, even on battlefields. I've heard them day and night—sometimes, I confess, I have been more asleep than awake. Some I've wanted to hear, some not—the "cocktail party consultation," the "restaurant recital," or the middle-of-the-night call from the "worried well." As a result of all this listening, however, one fact about illness has come to impress me more than any other: The perceived meanings and emotions contained in these tales are utterly crucial to their outcomes.

In the stories throughout this book I will use "meaning" in two ways. Sometimes I will refer to the meaning of a patient's illness—the patient's *interpretation* of the event; the *significance* it holds for him or her; what he or she believes it may symbolize, represent, or stand for. In this sense, meaning is akin to the "lesson" or the "message" embedded in illness that is extracted or gleaned by the person. The second way "meaning" is used is in examining the impact of "life meanings" on health and illness—the capacity of the perceived meanings and experiences of a lifetime to affect our bodies. I think it will be clear from the context of the case history which nuance of meaning is operating. But in both usages, *meaning is inseparable from the actual thoughts, feelings, and emotions of the patients themselves.* Because "meaning" and "emotion" occupy a continuum, in some cases we will drift from discussing meaning to examining the impact of an emotion such as shame, despair, guilt, hope, trust, or love. Some readers may find this troubling, but these ambiguities are intentional, unavoidable, and, I feel, desirable.

As a single example, consider the way meaning and emotions are inseparably linked in the Black Monday syndrome discussed in Part I (page 62). This syndrome derives its name from the fact that more fatal heart attacks occur on Monday around 9 A.M.—the beginning of the workweek—than any other time of the week. This observation correlates with findings that the best predictor of a first heart attack is *not* any of the major risk factors (high blood pressure, high cholesterol, smoking, and diabetes mellitus), but rather, *job dissatisfaction*. In analyzing these findings, we cannot avoid asking the question, What does one's job *mean* to the patient—satisfaction, loathing, dread, a challenge, or something else; and how do these perceived meanings affect the body to contribute to heart attacks on Monday morning? Another valid question is, What does the heart attack that occurs on Black Monday *mean*? What does it symbolize or represent—job dissatisfaction, unhappiness, "something physical," or perhaps nothing at all? *However* meaning is approached, the answers are almost always laden with emotion.

I acknowledge the enormous conceptual and philosophical complexity of meaning, and I honor the efforts of philosophers to provide rigorous, clean analyses of it. No doubt the treatment given meaning in this book will appear superficial to professional philosophers, particularly the way I allow meaning to shade into "emotion" or "thought" or "feeling." But my defense is the stories themselves. As with Black Monday syndrome, when meaning appears as a factor in health it seems *always* to be clothed with emotion, thought, and feeling. Frank's case makes this clear. The pattern of his heartbeat on the cardiac monitor was not interpretable without taking both meaning and emotion into account.

As a further example, consider a case in which a patient who was highly allergic to penicillin was given a placebo pill, an inert substance with no known biological effect. After he swallowed it he was told an untruth—that the pill was not a placebo but penicillin. The man immediately became fearful, experienced an anaphylactic ("allergic shock") reaction, and abruptly died. This was a genuine "death from meaning," for all that was manipulated in this situation was what the pill he had ingested *meant* to him. It has similarly been shown that persons can be provoked into allergy attacks on being shown a *picture* of a hayfield or *fake* flowers to which they are sensitive—again, reactions mediated by perceived meanings and not due to exposure to the "real thing."

Meaning exerts positive effects on health as well as negative ones. For example, during a coronary artery bypass operation on the heart, a hospital-wide power failure occurred just after the surgeon opened the chest by cutting through the sternum. Rather than continue under the risky conditions of the backup emergency power system, he aborted the operation. Even though no actual surgery on the heart was done, the patient was not told this, and the procedure continued to mean to her "the real thing." The operation proved to be a complete success: the crippling heart pain, angina pectoris, for which the surgery was done, went away completely.[13]

Cases such as these are often dismissed pejoratively as examples of the "placebo response," as if calling something "just a placebo" renders it unimportant and minimizes any effect of perceived meaning. It hardly matters; the man succumbing to what the placebo pill *meant* to him is not less dead because the placebo response was involved instead of penicillin.

It is not just in orthodox medicine that the vital role of meaning is overlooked. Sometimes those health workers who most vigorously advocate treating the "whole person" seem the most likely to neglect the importance of meaning. One can, for instance, find numerous "alternative" or "holistic" health books replete with tables and formulae purporting to show that a physical problem in a particular part of the body reflects a psychological problem in the patient's past—lack of parental love, child abuse, poor self-esteem, and an array of other deficiencies in nurturance and upbringing. Conversely, sometimes certain psychological events are predicted to cause specific illnesses in the future. While it is true beyond reasonable doubt that one's psychological and physical states are related, the relationships can be quite complex and impossible to describe by linear, invariant formulas that apply equally to all persons. What is left out of these simplistic notions, among other things, is the unique, individual, and idiosyncratic nature of meaning.

Because identical happenings in two different persons' lives may mean different things to each of them, it is *impossible in principle* to make rigid, uniform connections between life events and physical illness. Consider, for example, two married, middle-aged women with arteriosclerotic heart disease. Both learned their husbands were suing for divorce. One of the women experienced a cardiac arrest and died from the emotional shock. The other was jubilant that she would be freed finally from an unsatisfactory marriage. Her heart disease improved, her physician discontinued all her medications, and she took up a jogging program she had abandoned ten years earlier. For these women the event—learning of an impending divorce—was identical; but the different meaning contained in the event made all the difference. These cases show what is often forgotten: if attempts to connect life events and illness omit the all-important factor of meaning, they are doomed to failure. The linguist Alfred Korzybski effectively summed up this situation: "When a symbolic class of life enters the arena, hold your hats. All bets are off."[14]

"Is your health excellent, good, fair, or poor?" According to several studies done over the past few years, the answer people give to this simple question is a better predictor of who will live or die over the next decade than in-depth physical examinations and extensive laboratory tests. This question is a way of asking what our health *means* to us—what it represents or symbolizes in our thoughts and imagination—and is an example of the vital interplay between meaning and matter.

The best study of the impact of people's opinions on their health involved more than 2,800 men and women aged 65 and older conducted by sociologist Ellen Idler of Rutgers University and Stanislav Kasl of the Department of Epidemiology and Public Health at Yale Medical School.[15] Their findings are consistent with the results of five other large studies involving more than 23,000 people, ages 19 to 94. All these studies lead to the same conclusion: Our own opinion about the state of our health is a better predictor than objective factors such as physical symptoms, extensive exams and laboratory tests, or behaviors such as cigarette smoking. For instance, people who smoked were twice as likely to die over the next twelve years as people who did not, whereas those who say their health is "poor" are *seven* times more likely to die than those who say their health is "excellent."

Researchers point out, however, that these findings do not mean that people can "wish" their medical fate. Neither do they indicate that one's health is necessarily excellent just because one believes it to be so. Something could still be wrong, so there remains a place for physical exams and tests. These findings do suggest, however, that something else besides physical findings at the time of an exam are playing a role in who lives and dies, and that physicians should pay attention to what patients believe about their health, i.e., what their health *means* to them.[16]

Why should our perceived meanings of our health outperform in-depth physical exams and lab tests as long-term predictors of who lives and dies? Researchers don't know, but several theories have been offered. One possibility is that people take into account more factors than the physicians who are doing the exams and tests. For instance, a patient may be extremely mindful of the way he has cared for or neglected his health in the past, which may be unknown to the doctor. Another possibility is that beliefs act as self-fulfilling prophecies. If people believe their health is going to be played out in a certain way, they may act in ways that make these beliefs come true, "living out" their meanings and perceptions and translating them into the flesh. For example, if every male in my family has died before age 40 of a heart attack, I may expect the same fate and tailor my behavior accordingly. I may take a "what's the use?" attitude, smoke, and ignore dietary and exercise precautions and thus cooperate in having my heart attack on schedule. Third, people may have a delicate sense of an approaching illness based on subtle body cues such as fatigue, exhaustion, or diminished vitality and energy, which do not show up on physical exams and lab tests. As psychologist Howard Leventhal of Rutgers University put it, "It's clear that people are in some way aware of a general report from the body that things are or are not up to par."[17] These bodily feelings might act to generate particular meanings and expectations: "Something isn't right, something dreadful is about to happen." This apprehension, in turn, may lead to mood changes such as depression, or to changes in behavior such as isolation and restriction of healthful activities. The patient would then be caught in a "meaning loop" wherein body-based perceptions lead to certain meanings, which lead to unhealthy behaviors and moods, which create further bodily changes and worsening meanings, and on and on.[18]

Remove the meaning from patients' stories and they become unrecognizable—sanitized, dull, dry, as if they were being recited by a computer. This is why meaning accounts for the crucial difference between "disease" and "illness." Illness is something that happens to persons, while disease is what happens to organs of the body. Illness is disease plus meaning. When physicians forget about meaning, they are apt to believe they are treating only a disease, and they may actually begin to refer to their patient as such—"the heart attack in Room 4" or "the compound fracture in the Emergency Room."

The use of computers in medical practice has taught us a lot about meaning. In recent years frequent attempts have been made to employ them in obtaining case histories and making diagnoses. In one research project the computer could not match the diagnostic skills of seasoned physicians. The researchers were puzzled, since both the computer and the physicians asked the same questions and the patients gave the same answers to both. Why did the diagnoses differ? Trying to understand how the reasoning of the physicians differed from that of the computer, the researchers asked the physicians, "What is the first thing you notice in the interview?" The physicians replied, "Whether or not the patient is *sick*." Yet when pressed, they could not explain what "sick" meant. As all good diagnosticians know, it is a feeling, an intuition, a sense about whether something is genuinely wrong. It is something one detects from a *person,* not an organ. "Being sick" is manifested in subtle nuances of communication—body language, facial expressions, inflections of speech, even silence. It may be revealed as worry, concern, denial, fear, or pain. It is the outward expression of the inner meaning of the illness for the patient.

The physicians were able to "catch the meaning" of the patient's experience, the computer could not. Because meaning is impossible to quantify, the computer researchers could not discover ways to program it into the computer. As they discovered, the medical endeavor can fall flat when meaning is missed: a correct diagnosis can be impossible and appropriate therapy delayed.

When the meaning and significance of a health event for a patient are not sensed by a physician, the patient is usually the first to know. He may feel that "Dr. Jones is a fine doctor, but he's only interested in my heart; he really doesn't care about *me*." The patient is stating that Dr. Jones is behaving like the computer, unable to catch the meaning, significance, and importance of the problem to the person possessing it.

It is no use, in my judgment, arguing that disease means nothing. One can insist that it *should* mean nothing, as Susan Sontag has eloquently done in her influential book *Illness as Metaphor*,[19] but this is a hopeless ideal. Anyone who is seriously sick will find or create meaning to explain what is happening. It is simply our nature to do so, and I have never seen an exception to this generalization. Even if we *claim* that our illness means nothing, as did Sontag in her experience with cancer, we are creating and inserting meaning into the event. Here the meaning takes the form of denial—the denial of any underlying significance, purpose, or pattern—which is meaning of a negative kind. But *negative* meaning is not the same thing as *no* meaning. We may tell ourselves that our illness is nothing more than an accidental, purposeless, random event, that it is simply a matter of our atoms and molecules just being themselves. But this denial of meaning is meaning in disguise: It can assure us, for example, right or wrong, that the illness was not our fault, that we were not responsible for it, that it "just happened"—which can be a great consolation. Thus, negative meaning is extremely meaning*ful*.

One can, of course, rightly argue that in any given illness we may have extracted an incorrect meaning, drawn the wrong lesson, made an erroneous interpretation, become confused about what the illness represents, or misinterpreted the role our life meanings may have played in its genesis. But to deny totally the existence of meaning in illness is a position I find baffling. It has, of course, long been fashionable in science to deny a meaning behind existence in general, and this has affected medicine: if all of existence is meaningless, so, too, must disease be meaningless. Yet there is something extraordinarily ironic, if not oxymoronic, about impassioned essays advocating the meaninglessness of *anything*, including illness. As Whitehead wryly put it, "Scientists, animated by the purpose of proving they are purposeless, constitute an interesting subject for study."[20] The same holds, I feel, for doctors or patients who vigorously espouse the meaninglessness of health and illness. I am reminded of an observation by the physicist Niels Bohr: "The one certain thing is that a statement like 'existence is meaningless' is itself devoid of any meaning."

People *can* have a *sense* of meaninglessness. They genuinely may believe there is no meaning to their existence, including whatever illnesses they may develop.[21] They may deny vehemently that their perceived meanings affect their health, certain as they are that they themselves *have* no meaning. These protests are hollow, however, as the Swiss psychologist C. G. Jung knew. Toward the end of his life he said, "Meaninglessness . . . is . . . equivalent to illness."[22] Put another way: illness *is* the meaning of meaninglessness, as many of the following stories show.

How does meaning actually change the body? Today we know a great deal about the biochemical changes that follow perceptions, emotions, and meanings of various sorts. We know, for example, that the person who drops dead on hearing bad news does so because of sudden changes taking place in the autonomic nervous system—dilation of peripheral blood vessels, a fall in blood pressure, a dramatic slowing or standstill of the heart, or a cardiac arrhythmia. We know a lot about the sometimes fatal changes that take place in bereaved spouses in their first year of grief and depression, such as alterations in the function of immune cells that normally protect them from infections and cancer. We also know a lot about "positive biology"—physiological changes associated with hope, love, and optimism. Consequently we may believe we understand how meaning enters the body and actually changes it. Yet these explanations are largely an *illusion* of understanding and a failure to appreciate the subtleties involved. In fact, the fundamental mystery of *how* thought and perception gain access to the body remains largely untouched by the insights of modern science.

The interaction of mind and matter and the way in which meaning affects the body involve the so-called mind-body problem, one of the most difficult questions in the history of Western philosophy. How can a thought, which seems and "feels" nonphysical, alter cells, tissues, and organs, which seem overwhelmingly physical? How can such dissimilar things affect each other? It has never been clear to most persons who have thought deeply about this question how the actual interaction between atoms and thought takes place. When the mind affects the body it is as if some sort of magic has transpired, permitting material stuff somehow to be quickened by the mind.

Currently, one cannot even, as many health writers do, appeal to physics, our most accurate science, for a complete explanation of how mind and matter interact and how meaning, thought, and feeling affect the body. Two decades ago Nobel physicist Eugene Wigner summed up the inability of physics to solve the riddle of mind-body interaction, and his words still apply: "We have at present not even the vaguest idea how to connect the physico-chemical processes with the state of mind."[23]

If physics, our most accurate science, is in the dark about how consciousness interacts with matter, it is a gross exaggeration to say that medical science has explained how these processes take place. Medical science has, however, described many physical changes that correlate with the experience of certain meanings, thoughts, and emotions. Some of these correlations are known in considerable detail. As mentioned, today we can talk about the biology of hope, optimism, humor, depression, guilt, anxiety, fear, self-esteem, bereavement, or love. These correlations may involve not only major organs such as the heart or brain, but the activities of individual cells and molecules. Yet it is continually to be emphasized that these are *correlations* between mental and physical states, *not explanations* of how the interactions occur. They are a "what," not a "how"; they simply tell us that what happens, happens.

Solving the mystery of mind-body interaction and the role of meaning in health will in my judgment require a qualitative leap in understanding. We have made such leaps before. Prior to Einstein's $E = mc^2$, the most famous equation in the history of science, we could not conceive that energy and matter could be interchangeable and that they are related to each other by a third thing, the speed of light. But today, in spite of the fact that matter still *appears* completely different from energy—a pound of plutonium bears no resemblance to the mushroom cloud of a nuclear blast—we accept that there is an equivalence between the two. We have a new *feel* for the relationship of matter and energy, a new way of "being conscious" regarding this connection.

As with energy and matter, mind and matter may be equivalent even though they appear completely different. And just as energy and matter are related through a third entity, the speed of light, mind and matter also may be related through a third entity, *meaning*. Indeed, the theory that mind and matter are bridged by meaning has been advanced by one of the world's leading theoretical physicists, David Bohm. Many believe that Bohm may possibly do for mind and matter what Einstein did for energy and matter: show that these two entities, apparently so disparate and immiscible, interpenetrate and become each other. This development would be of the utmost importance. It might allow mind and meaning to take their place alongside matter and energy as major factors in health and illness. If this occurred, the contention that health and illness are "all physical" would be turned upside down. For, if mind and matter were equivalent, one might as well say that health and illness are "all mental"—or that they are both physical and mental. Yet recognizing this equivalence would not prevent either mind or matter from appearing as relatively independent factors in health. Just as energy and matter manifest in certain situations as if they are different and unrelated (we experience a rock as matter if we hold it and as energy if we are hit by it), so, too, might the cause of an illness sometimes appear completely physical and sometimes completely mental.

I believe that understanding the interaction of mind, meaning, and matter ultimately must involve going beyond science to a fundamental shift in consciousness—to what Nobel geneticist Barbara McClintock called the development of "a feeling for the organism." This shift occurs commonly during illness as is apparent in many of the stories in this book. This is one reason why so many patients seem to understand deeply the role of meaning in the world. These patients experience the impact of meaning firsthand. As a result, the mind-body "problem" for them ceases to be a problem at all. Many emerge from their experience astonished that there should even be a question whether meanings, emotions, and thought affect the body. They have undergone a radical shift in awareness that science seems largely unable to grant. They have developed "a feeling for the organism."

I began this book as a bare-bones collection of clinical stories. I wanted only to show *that* meaning, thought, and emotion matter, not how or why—that they enter the body and sometimes make the difference in life and death. I wanted to let the patients' tales speak for themselves, with no superfluous commentary from me. If these manifestations of the mind are so important, why analyze or interpret the obvious? The answer, I've come to realize, is that so many people either do not understand, or downright disagree, that meaning, thought, and emotions are important. Indeed, legions of laboratory-confined researchers and scores of philosophers—people who have little if any actual contact with sick persons—deny any role whatsoever to meaning in health and illness. And almost unbelievably (to me), many physicians take the same position. Moreover, as we've noted, many patients for various reasons prefer to believe that "it's all physical." So, in an attempt to clarify and underscore the role of mind and meaning in the following tales, I have here and there inserted my own commentary, which I hope will not detract from the stories themselves.

The stories in Part I, "Breakdown," may at first seem negative or even depressing to the reader. Perhaps this is inevitable; after all, these are the stories we physicians hear day after day; people do not make appointments to tell us how *well* they are doing. But although many of these tales are grim, that is not the whole of it. If one enters them imaginatively and empathically, trying genuinely to take the patient's point of view, the grimness hopefully will be outweighed by the awesome complexity of human existence that is revealed. We are witnessing here not just illness and disease but *life,* and the power of perceived meanings, attitudes, thoughts, and emotions to shape that life.

In Part II, "New Meaning, New Body," we propose a radically different image of the body: that it is not a machine, as we have been told, but *music,* down to the actual atoms and molecules that comprise it. A new picture emerges: *The body as an enchanted instrument on which mind and meaning play.* The metaphor of the musical body, we shall see, is not only consistent with certain spiritual insights that have developed through the ages, but also has been put forward by serious scientists.

The melodies flowing from the musical body are the "Healing Breakthroughs" that are the theme of Part III. Here the bright and triumphant side of meaning surfaces, and we see how the various manifestations of our consciousness can lead to greater health and wisdom. We will see that healing often is not the mechanical, physical process we generally believe it to be, not just a matter of having physical exams and tests, taking medications, or having surgery. Genuine healing is frequently unexpected and radical, seemingly out of the blue, and often depends not on what we *do* but on how we choose to *be*. The role of belief, hope, prayer, and the miraculous are examined, along with evidence for a benevolent, invisible healing force within each of us. We shall see that the physical does not always have the last word, and that even the manifestations of genetic diseases can yield to the power of the belief system.

LARRY DOSSEY, M.D.
Santa Fe, New Mexico

PART ONE

BREAKDOWN

The man who regards his own life and that of his fellow creatures as meaningless is not merely unhappy but hardly fit for life.

—ALBERT EINSTEIN[1]

The lack of meaning in life is a soul-sickness whose full extent and full import our age has not as yet begun to comprehend.

—C. G. JUNG[2]

The Asthmatic and the Intern:
When Shame Is Fatal

"Where do you want me to start? From the beginning of my troubles?" Jennie spoke easily at first to the doctor conducting the interview.

"Yes, of course," the young physician replied. He was an intern at Los Angeles County General Hospital, in his first year of training after receiving his M.D. degree. He knew Jennie was twenty-seven years old, was experiencing great difficulty with asthma, and had an extraordinarily chaotic life.

"When I was a child we lived in Arkansas," Jennie continued. "My mother was quite religious and brought us up in the Baptist faith. I have never known my father and nobody knew his whereabouts. To tell the truth, I think my parents never were married at all.

"When I went to school I made some money as a baby-sitter. The baby's mother was always good to me, better than my own mother, and when I moved to California later on she still used to send me checks occasionally. I came to Los Angeles at the age of seventeen, and at first my asthma improved quite a bit."

"Did you move to California because of your health?" the doctor inquired.

"Well, this was not the only reason, but must I tell you all those things?" Jennie was obviously troubled about revealing the details of her past.

"Certainly," the physician assured her. "You should relieve your mind by speaking about everything that happened in those days." The intern had learned one of his lessons well, that only by "getting it out" can the pain of past experiences be addressed. He was pushing Jennie for a full disclosure.

"Back in the little town in Arkansas a man fooled me into an affair and I became pregnant. When the child was born my mother was very mad at me and behaved terribly. I never heard any kind words from her. I had the feeling that she wanted to get rid of me and the child."

"What about the father of the child?" the doctor wanted to know.

"He was no good," Jennie responded. "He threatened to kill me if I ever revealed his name to anyone as the father of the child. He even told me he would come to Los Angeles to kill me if I did so. For that reason I never dared to ask for help from any state agency. The only one helping me with money was the lady from my home town once in a while, so I was able to register in junior college. To make ends meet I stayed with my two brothers who had come to Los Angeles and found jobs."

"Did you finish junior college?"

By this time, Jennie was becoming very agitated and nervous. "No, I did not," she said. "I had to quit because I could not stay with my brothers any longer."

"Why?" the doctor persisted.

"Do I have to tell you that, too?" Jennie asked, extremely anxious.

"Certainly, you should," he said. "You have no reason to be ashamed of anything." The physician would not yield in his honesty-is-the-best-policy approach.

"It was impossible for me to live with my brothers," Jennie reluctantly revealed. She had begun to weep. "One of them frequently made advances at me and even tried to rape me." She was now very excited. "So I moved to a single apartment on county aid. Since I had to make a living, I quit junior college and took occasional domestic jobs."

"What about your asthma?"

"Oh, it became much worse at that time," Jennie responded excitedly. "I frequently had to be admitted to the hospital for a few days of treatment. This meant that I would always lose my job. I have no hope anymore of recovering. That's why I wanted to die, and want to die now all the time—because I am no good, no good!"

By now Jennie was severely agitated and profoundly short of

breath. She reached for her Isuprel nebulizer, an inhalation device used for acute symptoms of asthma. As she did so she experienced a generalized seizure with violent contractions and spasms involving her entire body. She rapidly became unconscious. In spite of intensive emergency medical treatment, Jennie never regained awareness. She died within a few minutes after stating she wanted to die and being pressured into reliving the shameful events of her life.[1]

When I first read about Jennie's tragic case, I immediately recalled one of my own patients whose sense of shame, guilt, and personal failure almost proved fatal.

Responding to the 3:00 A.M. phone call from the emergency room physician, I found Carol, a patient of mine of many years, lying on a stretcher. In her mid-thirties and very health conscious, she came to my office only for routine checkups. She prided herself on being completely self-sufficient in matters of health, and attributed her success to positive attitudes and a healthy lifestyle that included a variety of alternative methods of health care. But now she was near death—unable to talk coherently and with a temperature of 104° F., a falling blood pressure, and a rapid pulse. Her examination showed a rigid, painful abdomen, usually a sign of inflammation or infection. Intravenous fluids and antibiotics were begun immediately, and following some simple blood tests and X rays of her abdomen, Carol was taken to surgery. She had a ruptured appendix. Her recovery was prolonged and complicated but eventually complete.

I was puzzled that she had waited until the advanced stages of appendicitis before seeking my help. Persons with appendicitis usually have lots of warning signs before the appendix ruptures—especially pain in the right lower abdomen, sometimes for days—signs that are well known to most people. During her recovery, Carol hesitantly revealed the sequence of events. Interested as ever in preventive measures and personal responsibility, she tried several ways of treating her problem when the pains began. These included a special diet and a variety of medications that had been recommended by friends as a "natural" therapy for "inflammation." When they did not work and the pain increased, she sought acupuncture treatments, which helped temporarily.

Her illness gathered steam, however, and soon the fever began. She tried several other alternative therapies, to no avail.

"But why didn't you call me? Why did you wait until you nearly died?" I asked. Carol had begun to weep.

"Because I was so ashamed!"

Through her tears, Carol described her belief that all illness is somehow connected with the mind, which meant to her that she had a hand in creating her problem in the first place. She thus wanted to deal with it in her own ways, ways that lay outside modern medicine. When her methods failed she began to feel guilty about her unorthodox choices, and she chose to suffer in silence rather than sound the alarm. She did not want to come to my office and have to "confess" her methods and reveal her failure. It was apparent that she feared my disapproval, which I found very troubling.

"Why not use both approaches?" I asked. "Why paint yourself into a corner? Why not feel free to use whatever works?"

Carol's experience was therapeutic for both of us. For her it was a chance to expand her concepts of the origins of health and illness, and how to manage when things go wrong. For me it was a stimulus to ask myself difficult and painful questions. Why was my own patient ashamed to come to my office when she failed? Why would she rather risk death than disapproval? Had I unwittingly contributed to her problem? For both of us, the answers continue to evolve.

There are thousands of Carols—persons who prefer unconventional, simple, "natural," or "holistic" methods to those offered by orthodox physicians, and who experience a sense of personal failure, shame, and guilt when things go wrong. Too often the response of physicians to such a person is condescending and judgmental, which only increases whatever guilt and shame the person may experience if the methods don't work out.

But patients taking the unorthodox path largely are not the uneducated, naive, and irresponsible persons that physicians often consider them to be. In a study of 660 cancer patients, researcher Barrie Cassileth and her colleagues at the University of Pennsylvania Cancer Center found this stereotype to be wrong. They discovered that persons seeking unorthodox cancer treatments were in fact better educated than those seeking orthodox treatment only. Nor were these persons, as is often thought, desperate, end-stage patients who had exhausted conventional treatments. The majority tended to think their cancer was preventable, that chemotherapy and radiation were harmful or useless, and that unorthodox therapies—diet, megavitamins, imagery, "spiritual" methods, and others—were more helpful. This study also found misleading the stereotype of the unorthodox practitioner as a charlatan or quack. Sixty percent were well-trained physicians (M.D.s) who did not charge high fees.[2]

In her remarkable, insightful book, *Guilt Is the Teacher, Love Is the Lesson,* psychobiologist Dr. Joan Borysenko distinguishes between unhealthy and healthy guilt. Unhealthy guilt is the kind experienced by Jennie and Carol. This type of guilt can literally be channeled into the body and cause death, as Jennie's case shows. The person thinks of himself or herself as utterly unworthy, and when anything goes wrong, immediately resorts to self-blame. And, like Jennie, he or she can go a step further and assume that "it's always going to be this way" and "there's nothing I can do about it."

Unhealthy guilt is closely connected with feelings of shame. "Shame feels like a sudden severing of our connection with the world," Borysenko states. "It leaves us feeling emotionally . . . naked. . . . Shame is shockingly painful and isolating. [It] is the absolute picture of helplessness. We are beaten and we know it."[3] Again, Jennie's and Carol's experiences with illness are classic examples.

What about healthy guilt? Psychologist Blair Justice, in his valuable book *Who Gets Sick: Thinking and Health* describes how healthy guilt operates. Suppose a person discovers his checking account is overdrawn. Unhealthy guilt would prompt him to say, "I'm incapable of doing anything right." A healthier response might be to consider that perhaps the bank had made a mistake—"All banks make errors"—or to make allowances for special circumstances—for example, "I've been sick with the flu for a week; I've let everything slide, including balancing my checkbook."[4] Healthy guilt does not hide from the facts—the checkbook *is* unbalanced—but it does not require the person to "beat himself up" with inappropriate blame and recrimination, and it does not lead to shame.

Most importantly, healthy guilt can be used as a springboard for responsible action and continued growth and change. This is illustrated in the case of Anna, a patient of Dr. Shelley E. Taylor's, professor of psychology at UCLA and author of *Positive Illusions*.[5]

Anna was a lovely woman in her mid-fifties. Both she and her husband had practiced a healthy lifestyle, long before it was popular to do so. Both prided themselves in rarely being sick, having missed between them only two days of work in nearly fifteen years. Thus, when Anna was diagnosed with breast cancer, both were upset. They felt invulnerable to disease, and there was no history of breast cancer in Anna's family. At first the shock was debilitating, but shortly after surgery Anna began to fight back. In spite of the fact that her faith in diet and exercise had been shaken, she continued to believe that these were her best weapons in fighting cancer. She therefore threw herself back into her health program with renewed enthusiasm—increasing her running, eliminating red meat altogether, and making additional alterations in her diet. Then her cancer recurred.

By the time Dr. Taylor interviewed her for the first time, her efforts to control her body had failed dramatically, not once but twice. Dr. Taylor asked how she had responded when the recurrence developed in spite of her renewed efforts at good health.

"She shrugged and said she guessed she'd been wrong," Dr. Taylor reported. "She did not abandon her healthy lifestyle, but rather decided to redirect her energies in a new direction. She quit her dull job and used her remaining time to write short stories—something she had always wanted to do. Having lost control in one area of her life, she turned to another area, her work life, that was still controllable."

Anna's is a classic example of healthy guilt in action. Although she admitted being wrong, she did not withdraw into doing nothing. She was not paralyzed by endless self-recrimination, and her realization of being wrong did not progress to shame. Each setback gave her insight on which to build a new plan of action.

Persons paralyzed by shame are usually examples of "learned helplessness." This concept was developed by psychologist Martin Seligman and his colleagues at the University of Pennsylvania. Beginning in the 1960s they discovered that when dogs were administered unavoidable, inescapable shocks, eventually they just seemed to give up. Even when given a chance to escape—by being moved to a different cage with only a low barrier over which they could jump—they acted helpless and continued to accept the shocks. In other experiments, if animals were exposed to the shocks but *from the start* had the chance to escape them, they did not learn to give up and become helpless. These studies seemed to indicate that it was the *perception of control* that was paramount. The theory was eventually extended to people as well. If we are repeatedly in situations we *believe* are beyond our control, we expect our actions to be totally useless in changing our situation. These feelings can eventually progress to a pervasive sense of unworthiness, guilt, and shame.

When people learn, like Jennie, to be genuinely helpless, they tend chronically to react to their problems with the classic triad of "I caused it," "It'll always be this way," and "This is going to spoil everything else I do." This point of view seems actually to be channeled into the body. It creates physiological changes that set the stage for bad health. When Seligman and his colleagues rated 172 undergraduates for the presence or absence of this explanatory style, they accurately *predicted* which students would be sick the most; the predictions held both one month and one year later. In another study involving 13 patients who had malignant melanoma, absence of this style of explanation was a better predictor of survival than even the level of activity of natural killer cells, a type of white blood cell crucial in the immune response.[6]

Jennie's case of fatal asthma shows that the lungs can be the target organ for internalized guilt and shame. The cases in the following chapter illustrate perhaps the commonest victim: the heart.

Caught in the Act:
Forbidden Play and Cardiac Arrest

It was a day that would change forever the life of this healthy thirty-nine-year-old teacher. Roughhousing in the den with his two teenage daughters, he heard the doorbell suddenly ring. Without hesitation, one of the daughters got up from the floor to answer it. When the unannounced visitor, a neighbor, appeared at the door of the room and witnessed the frolicsome scene, the startled father looked up and exclaimed, "I'm sorry," and instantly fell over with cardiac arrest.

Fortunately the man's wife was a registered nurse and began immediately to administer CPR (cardiopulmonary resuscitation). An ambulance was called and the emergency technicians continued resuscitation measures while transporting the man to a community hospital. Here he was found to be in ventricular fibrillation, a chaotic pattern of heartbeat that is uniformly fatal if not promptly corrected. He was eventually defibrillated with great difficulty, was "hooked up" in the coronary care unit, and within twelve hours had regained consciousness.

Although his life had been saved and tests showed that he apparently had not sustained a heart attack, his problems were far from over. He continued to have life-threatening cardiac arrhythmias despite the use of potent drugs to suppress them. Because he was not responding to treatment, on the twentieth day following his collapse he was transferred to the Peter Bent Brigham Hospital at Harvard Medical School for further evaluation and therapy.

While in the coronary care unit at the Harvard hospital, the man continued to demonstrate frequent life-threatening cardiac arrhythmias.

On the sixth night following his transfer he was restless and expressed some vague premonitions. Although he fell asleep readily at 10:30 and appeared to sleep peacefully, at 4:00 A.M. he experienced another episode of ventricular fibrillation. This was dealt with immediately by the coronary care unit nurses.

The man was subjected to every cardiac diagnostic test available at Harvard Medical School that might shed light on his problem. They were all normal, and no specific disease entity could be proved. These findings were of little consolation to him: although "normal," he had almost died twice and was still having problems.

The life-threatening abnormalities of his heartbeat were particularly prevalent when emotionally upsetting events would occur—as when his psychologist would enter the room. These associations became so obvious that a decision was finally made to try to deal definitively with them.

The man underwent four psychiatric interviews and several psychological tests. During his interviews he seemed defensive and hyperalert, despite his languid, folksy manner. He demonstrated strong emotional undercurrents of hostility and competition, was loquacious, and resisted interruptions. He repeatedly denied having depressive or angry thoughts, and in spite of his recent cardiac arrest he dismissed any fear.

A central pattern of his life was controlled aggression. He grew up in a tough mining town, was intensely competitive with his one brother, and had overcome enormous obstacles in obtaining higher education. He expended fierce energy in every enterprise. He had dedicated his life as a teacher to helping others and promoting brotherhood. He frequently found himself boiling with anger, which he sought to neutralize with vigorous solitary exercise. He made it his habit to avoid violent television programs, yet violence erupted frequently in his dreams, a symptom he disowned as not part of his true self.

Equally strong were his moral prohibitions regarding sexuality. Deeply religious, he insisted that his only sexual thoughts were for his wife, even though his work involved close contact with many other women in his community. Yet the roughhousing with his daughters just prior to his cardiac arrest had aroused strong erotic impulses in him, his interviewers found.

In an attempt to calm the emotional storms brewing inside him, the man was taught to meditate. An instructor in the famous TM (Transcendental Meditation) technique came to his bedside and instructed him in clearing his mind and calming his body. Meditation was carried out for twenty minutes twice a day.

The results were impressive. He would sit in front of his cardiac monitor and try to subdue through meditation the ventricular premature beats as they would arise on the screen. After a week he became quite skillful at this. On several occasions when he was harboring a great deal of emotional tension and was starting to exhibit advanced grades of arrhythmias, he was able to eradicate these disturbing patterns at will.

With the complementary use of meditation and cardiac drugs, he recovered and left the hospital. In addition to continuing both meditation and medication, he was particularly encouraged to verbalize his dreams, even when their content was violent, loathsome, or shameful.

The approach was enormously successful. At last report he is still well and continues to jog several miles a day. [1]

This young man's case vividly shows that the anxiety, shame, and guilt surrounding forbidden sexual acts can be an emotional witches' brew that is toxic to the heart. Like Jennie above, this man's confrontation with death came with a sudden, overwhelming sense of shame, which he acknowledged with what almost proved to be his final words, "I'm sorry."

It is not just incestuous acts that set these events in motion. Other socially forbidden sexual behaviors appear to do the same. One such is bigamy, a criminal offense. There is evidence that bigamy, like incest or rape, can trigger sudden death. Doctors Martin S. Gizzi and Bernard Gitler, of New Rochelle Hospital Medical Center, have proposed "the contemplation of bigamy" as an outright risk factor for death from coronary artery disease, along with high cholesterol, high blood pressure, smoking, and diabetes. They report two typical cases:

A fifty-three-year-old man who had undergone coronary artery bypass surgery eleven years before was admitted to the hospital with chest pain thought to represent a heart attack. On the morning after he was admitted, his wife visited him in the coronary care unit. Shortly after she left another woman arrived, to whom he had become engaged. Following her departure the man died from cardiac arrest.

A previously healthy thirty-four-year-old man was admitted to the coronary care unit with severe chest pain representing a massive heart attack. He subsequently developed ventricular fibrillation but was successfully resuscitated. The morning after being stabilized he was visited by his fiancée. That same afternoon he was visited by another woman also claiming to be his fiancée.

Gizzi and Gitler suggest that, in the latter case, the man's chaotic sexual life may have been a primary factor in his brush with death from heart disease.

"We were struck by the youth of the patients, the severity of their disease, and the singular nature of their emotional predicament," these researchers state. "We propose that multiple spouses or fiancées may present such severe psychological stress as to accelerate the course of coronary artery disease, thereby qualifying as a new risk factor not previously identified."[2]

The catastrophic consequences that can accompany forbidden sexual acts also surface in the lore of medical history. A singular example was reported by one of the greatest figures in the history of Western medicine, Giovanni Battista Morgagni (1682–1771). Morgagni was a distinguished professor at Padua, and he lay the foundation of modern pathology as a true science. He was one of the first persons to describe the rupture of an aortic aneurysm, an outpouching or enlargement of the body's largest blood vessel. Here is his graphic account, first published in the English language in 1769:

A strumpet of eight-and-twenty years of age, of a lean habit, having complain'd for some months, and particularly for the last fifteen days, of a certain lassitude, and a loathing of food, and almost of everything, for this reason made less use of other aliments and more of unmix'd wine; to the use of which she had always been too much addicted. A certain debauchee having gone into the house to her, and after a little time having come out, with a confus'd and disturb'd countenance and she not having appear'd for two or three hours after, the neighbours, who had observed these things, entering in, found her not only dead but cold;

lying in bed with such a posture of the body, that it could not be doubted what business she had been about when she died, especially as the semen verile was seen to have flow'd down from the organs of generation. . . . I conjectur'd . . . that the cause of this sudden death would certainly be found to consist in the rupture of some large vessel.[3]

Morgagni's speculation was right on target, as his autopsy of the promiscuous "strumpet" confirmed.

This patient had a predisposing physical abnormality that was a factor in her sudden death, an aneurysm of the aorta; thus, her case is hardly typical. But even in the general population, illicit sex continues to be a factor in sudden death. In one well-known study, in which death during sexual activity accounted for 0.6 percent of sudden deaths from internal causes, most of these occurred in the setting of extramarital intercourse. Men were on average thirteen years older than their companions, and one-third were inebriated at the time of intercourse.[4] Purely physical explanations have been offered for these findings. It has been suggested that the demands on the cardiovascular system are greater during extramarital intercourse than during sex with a marital companion of a lifetime—the effects of novelty, titillation, fantasy, excitement, and heightened physical activity. Thus it might be expected that sudden death rates would be higher during extramarital sex. But in view of the specific case histories above involving forbidden acts—the guilt-ridden young teacher who experienced cardiac arrest after erotically roughhousing with his daughters, and the heart attack victims who apparently were affected by "the contemplation of bigamy"—we can wonder if shame and guilt do not also play a role in sudden deaths during extramarital sex, in addition to whatever physical factors may be present.

"Shame is innate," Dr. Joan Borysenko states. "We don't learn how to be ashamed. It is 'factory installed.'"[5] But if so, what was the reason for the installation? Evolutionary theory suggests that our capacity to "be shamed" should have survival value, otherwise it would not have developed so conspicuously in the evolutionary ascent of humans. Could shame have a higher purpose, a positive value?

We've already seen that shame and guilt can be a stimulus for positive change—Borysenko's concept of "healthy guilt" illustrated in Anna's experience with breast cancer. Additionally, most people believe that we *should* feel shameful and guilty if we've committed certain acts, such as hurting others. In these instances guilt and shame serve to steer us back to an appropriate course of behavior. These positive effects operate at a societal and cultural level. In addition, there may be another valuable side to these emotions—one that can be lifesaving and is shared with a great variety of other creatures.

When animals are shamed, they behave in a typical way. They tend to cower, slink, or become immobile. They appear to withdraw deeply into themselves and retreat, as if expecting the worst. Most persons can recall finding themselves in similar situations—moments during which, in Borysenko's words, "we are beat and we know it." This behavior is quite similar to the "freeze" reaction to crisis, described by UCLA psychiatrists Lizzy Jarvik and Dan Russell. The freeze response is a "wait and see" behavior, a stopping of all voluntary action in an attempt to weather a storm. Like the physical response to shame, it allows breathing room and a time for the threatening situation to improve. It is a particularly optimal strategy, Jarvik and Russell suggest, for people with declining resources such as the very young, the elderly or weak, or those who are very ill.

All organisms use inactivity as a means of coping. The amoeba contracts and ceases to move if a stimulus is too intense, and if the stimulus is protracted, will remain immobile until death. Doodlebugs curl up if challenged, and land turtles and tortoises retreat into their shells. Larger animals will hibernate, feign death, and demonstrate "tonic immobility" to cope with various stresses in their environment such as excessive heat or cold. Animals frequently "freeze" when captured by predators. This seems to be a valuable adaptation, as they are sometimes released unharmed. Humans, too, have been known to be released from the jaws of grizzlies on "going limp" and ceasing to struggle. In primates, the typical bodily position for this response seems to be sitting with the head tucked between the legs, with the arms pulled inward, supporting and protecting the face. Children dying of starvation assume this knee-chest position, and it can be seen not infrequently in adults following devastating events in which they feel totally helpless, such as earthquakes.[6]

Since this behavior also is seen in human beings undergoing the experience of overwhelming shame, we can speculate that intense shame may help us weather physical threats. From a biological perspective shame therefore would have survival value, and it would make sense that it became "factory installed" in the long course of evolution and is today "original equipment" at birth.

To withstand overwhelming shame human beings have also evolved another technique, which involves the ability of the personality or sense of "I" to fragment and multiply, literally to scatter when under attack.

Cases of multiple personality syndrome—among the most bizarre clinical tales ever recorded—are associated with the unendurable onslaught of shame early and repeatedly in life. Like the above stories, these tales, which we will now examine, are reminders that clinical problems are not "all physical." They represent prior happenings that cannot be entirely explained by what our atoms and molecules are doing—a meaning behind the disease.

The Siege of Shame:
The Multiple Personality Disorder

85 to 90 percent of MPD [multiple personality disorder] patients were beaten, cut, burned, half-drowned in bathtubs, locked in closets, hung out of windows, and/or sexually assaulted as children (generally before the age of ten), and their early histories are sagas of criticism, betrayal, abandonment, and inconsistency.

—JUDITH HOOPER AND DICK TERESI
The Three-Pound Universe[1]

"I am thirty-five years old and . . . a multiple. . . . I was molested a lot by my stepfather, and when I was six I was raped. My core personality went out then, at age six, and my host personality, Mary, took over.

"Only one person in my family knows. That's the case with most multiple personalities. You just don't see it if you're not looking for it. My first husband, poor dear, never knew what hit him.

"See, part of my personality went to sleep for a year and woke up married to Eddie—that's my ex-husband—and I could not tolerate him. Monica was the one who married him. What happened was that Mary's fiancé had drowned and when he drowned she konked out for a year. When she woke up married to Eddie she couldn't stand him. She also resented being thrown into this situation because she didn't know she was a multiple at the time. She didn't know that Monica existed."[2]

When Judith Hooper and Dick Teresi wrote a popular magazine article on MPD, multiple personality disorder, they received the above letter from a reader. The molestation and rape are typical of the abuse children experienced prior to the splitting of their self-identity into different personalities. Here is another example of the almost unbelievable agony these children endure: "A man buried his nine-year-old stepson alive, with a stovepipe over his face so he could breathe. The man then urinated through the pipe onto the boy's face."[3]

Psychobiologist Joan Borysenko describes the need of all children for trust:

> Trust is important to adults, but it is crucial for children because they have such a limited notion of how the world operates. Trust means that the world stays constant. . . . If Mommy praises Molly for picking up her toys today, Molly assumes that picking them up will please Mommy tomorrow. If rules change in midstream, the child's tenuous picture of "reality" collapses, and she will hold herself to blame for the painful feelings of confusion and shame that follow. . . . The interpersonal bridge is severed. . . . Feeling scared and isolated, the child wonders what she did to bring this disaster about. . . . To a small child who knows so little about the world, a fragile being whose life is totally dependent on parental care, broken bridges are as frightening as death. *The emotional response to the sudden collapse of reality that follows broken bridges is shame.*[4]

Childhood shame may result "only" in the development of distrust and suspicion about the world in general and a poor self-image and low esteem. But if the shame is the result of a situation in which the child is physically abused, tormented, and trapped, other ways of managing may surface. Psychiatrist Frank Putnam, of the National Institute of Mental Health and a leading authority on MPD, believes a basic coping strategy for severely abused children is "divide and conquer." "They cope with the pain and horror of the abuse," he states, "by dividing it up into little pieces and storing it in such a way that it's hard to put back together and hard to remember.[5] A form of self-hypnosis is probably involved. The child goes into trances, and that trance-state consciousness grows more and more autonomous and differentiated.[6] Eventually, various personalities come into play, perhaps analogous to the imaginary companions that normal children quite commonly have. These personalities can help shoulder the pain, and give children a way of distancing from it—allowing them to say, in effect, "This is not really happening to me, but to someone else." The number of personalities that emerge to help shoulder the pain seem limitless. A multiple may have hundreds of them, the average being thirteen.

Multiple personality disorder, states writer Edward Dolnick, can be viewed as an extreme form of "spacing out," not incorporating one's experiences into one's consciousness. Psychiatrists call this dissociation, and it is a quite normal reaction we all engage in to some degree, such as driving unconsciously on the freeway and having no memory for it. But in traumatic and painful events, dissociation goes a step further, not just in children but in adults as well. Bruno Bettelheim, who survived his experiences at Buchenwald and Dachau, recorded the experience he and his companions had on being forced to stand outside all night in temperatures so cold that twenty men died. "The prisoners did not care whether the SS shot them; they were indifferent to acts of torture. . . . It was as if what was happening did not 'really' happen to oneself. There was a split between the 'me' to whom it happened, and the 'me' who really did not care and was just a vaguely interested, but essentially detached, observer."[7]

As we will see so often in the case histories in this book, emotions do not stay in the mind; they spill into the body and metamorphose into a variety of physical manifestations. Nowhere is this more obvious than in the multiple, who can be a showcase of bizarre, seemingly inconsistent physical happenings:

One multiple has three menstrual periods every month, one for each of her identities. Others require different prescription glasses for their alter egos. A multiple can harbor one identity that knows how to drive and another that doesn't; one that speaks a foreign language fluently and another with a tin ear. Chicago psychiatrist Bennet Braun studied a man who was allergic to citrus drinks in all personalities but one. [Psychiatrist Frank] Putnam has met multiples who are actually married to two different people. . . . The repertoire of a multiple includes dramatic shifts in facial expression, accent, vocabulary, body language, clothing and hair styles, handwriting, phobias, and—above all—memories.[8]

Some skeptics think the multiple is "faking it," but this appears to have been disproved beyond doubt. At the National Institute of Mental Health, Daniel Weinberger has done cerebral blood flow studies in which the subject inhales radioactive xenon gas. There were radical differences between the blood flow patterns of different personalities.[9]

The violence that can occur between subpersonalities also makes it unlikely that the syndrome is a fake. Consider the following account reported by science writer Daniel Goleman in his book *Vital Lies, Simple Truths:*

The searing pain roused Marianna from sleep. She switched on the bedside light and saw dark red streaks of blood covering her sheets. She counted the fine lines of 30 razor cuts on her arms and legs before she carefully climbed out of bed. On her dresser was a note, written in childish scrawl:

WARNING TO MARIANNA
The lies must stop. Put a stop to the child or I'll kill.
—THE RIPPER

It was a death threat. But it was also a suicide attempt— for Marianna, the Child and the Ripper all inhabit the same body. The Ripper, a violent male personality given to fits of rage, felt angry and threatened because the Child, a youngster of four, had told their therapist the deeply hidden secrets the Ripper had guarded for so many years. His vicious attack was intended to make sure the Child stopped tattling. Never mind that he, the Child and Marianna all share the same body; they do not share the same pain. To the Ripper, they are different people, and he does not realize that death to the Child means death to him, too.[10]

MPD is a vivid demonstration of the ways that illness contains meaning. On one hand, the "meaning of life" for the multiple—life as pain, torment, confusion, and unpredictability—is the generative force for the emergence of the multiple personalities themselves. On the other hand, meaning presents itself in a somewhat different way to clinicians, who are looking on as outside observers. For clinicians, each case of MPD *has* a meaning, because it represents and symbolizes something beyond the physical or mental manifestations themselves. Although they may look at physical changes—the differences that exist between the multiple personalities—clinicians realize these are not the full story. Without taking into account what these changes *represent* and *symbolize,* clinicians cannot fully interpret them. And if they do not know what they *mean,* intelligent therapy becomes impossible. So the therapist cannot be content merely to focus on the physical events themselves, but must search for the meaning behind them. Only in uncovering the hidden meaning can he or she help restore wholeness to the patient.

It is dramatically obvious in MPD that denying the presence of meaning in illness leads to a watered-down practice of the art of medicine. Unless the hidden meanings are sought, therapy becomes a parody. What is gained by treating the allergic symptoms of one personality with an antihistamine, when ninety-nine more *nonallergic* personalities exist?

The shame and guilt that most persons experience are not as extreme as in the exotic MPD stories. We manage to weather the storms of childhood, emerging apparently with reasonably well-integrated, intact *single* personalities. But many skilled researchers of the human mind believe this may not be true. They tell us that we *all* may be multiples.

Psychiatrist Piero Ferrucci suggests we each are a patchwork, an arabesque of interwoven parts that usually work so harmoniously we never suspect their existence. The parts, however, are always there, functioning behind the scenes. In his important book *What We May Be,* he states:

> One of the most harmful illusions that can beguile us is probably the belief that we are an indivisible, immutable, totally consistent being. . . .
>
> Subpersonalities are psychological satellites, coexisting as a multitude of lives within the overall medium of our personality. Each subpersonality has a style and a motivation of its own, often strikingly dissimilar from those of the others. Says the Portuguese poet Fernando Pessoa, "In every corner of my soul there is an altar to a different god."
>
> Each of us is a crowd. There can be the rebel and the intellectual, the seducer and the housewife, the saboteur and the aesthete, the organizer and the bon vivant—each with its own mythology, and all more or less comfortably crowded into one single person. Often they are far from being at peace with one another. As Assagioli wrote, "We are not unified; we often feel that we are, because we do not have many bodies and many limbs, and because one hand doesn't usually hit the other. But, metaphorically, that is exactly what does happen within us. Several subpersonalities are continually scuffling: impulses, desires, principles, aspirations are engaged in an unceasing struggle."[11]

If this sounds depressing, it need not be. In fact, it may be a reason for optimism. It suggests that our conscious "I" does not always have to be on stage and in charge. Unknown to us, hidden aspects of the self look after us and shoulder part of the load.

Dr. Ernest Hilgard of Stanford University, a leading authority on hypnosis, has found that an aspect of the psyche he calls the "hidden observer" exists in just under half of all subjects who are highly hypnotizable. This entity exists, quite normally, completely outside conscious awareness, "looking on." And he finds that in quite normal people there can be overlapping cognitive control systems—multiple streams of consciousness—operating in everyday experience. Many contemporary researchers believe these multiple, hidden parts of ourselves may play a key role in creativity, healing, and other exceptional abilities.[12]

In MPD patients there seems to be an entity similar to the hidden observer. Psychiatrists Ralph Allison and Cornelia Wilber, pioneers in treating this problem, have called this the Inner Self Helper. It is a wise, benign, benevolent guide, unlike many of the alter personalities found in multiples. The Inner Self Helper seems to have no date of origin but appears to be timeless, "know[ing] the patient's past history and . . . predict[ing] future actions with great accuracy." It does not serve ordinary functions such as dealing with anger or sexuality, but appears dedicated to serving larger issues. It expects to work with the therapist, says Allison, and to "serve as a conduit for God's healing power and love."[13]

Many therapists working with MPD patients describe a consistent finding: the Inner Self Helper considers itself to be immortal. Under hypnosis, when the several alter personalities are asked what will happen to them when the body dies, they respond that they, too, will die. But a leading researcher in MPD, Dr. Jacqueline Damgaard, says that in contrast the Inner Self Helper declares that it shall remain forever. It seems to be the Eternal Self, saying, "I have always been."[14]

Shame is a great teacher about the role of meaning in our lives. The dramatic physical impact of shame shows that we literally *embody* the meanings we perceive in life's experiences, incorporating meaning into our organs and tissues as surely as water and food.

Now we look at an emotion with which shame keeps close company: despair.

F O U R

Halloween and Helplessness:
To Mean Nothing Is to Die

John was having a mastectomy. For a year he had endured the painful, foul-smelling abscesses in his right breast. So far, nothing had worked, neither the antibiotics nor the many surgical attempts to incise and drain the infected sites. The painful, oozing sores always recurred. He had been unable to work for most of the year and was fed up with the ordeal. He could not go on the way things were, and removing the breast seemed the only thing to do.

He decided to enter the hospital in August. The operation went smoothly, but in spite of the fact that he had no prior history of heart disease John had a heart attack the evening following surgery while recovering from anesthesia. He survived and eventually was discharged. On returning home, however, he became increasingly depressed. According to his wife, he was particularly disturbed that he could not return to work.

That Halloween, a group of local kids exploded fireworks in his mailbox, damaging it severely. When John surveyed the damage to his property, to which he was deeply attached, his wife said he became "not angry" but overwhelmed and utterly filled with despair. After all, he was recuperating from a heart attack, which prevented him from taking any action. John kept these feelings of despair inside, his typical way of coping.

Several days later his wife persuaded him to take the first stroll of his convalescence in their garden, hoping to cheer him up. As they ventured outside they noticed that an arbor, which John had built earlier that summer and of which he was very proud, had been sprayed with black tar paint by the Halloween pranksters. John was again overwhelmed and stared helplessly at his beloved construction while his wife fumed and expressed her anger. Then he remarked that he did not feel well and wished to return to the house. He turned, walked twenty yards, and collapsed. As he did so, his wife asked if he was experiencing pain, and he said no.

Within five minutes he was dead.

Later on, John's physicians interviewed his wife. They wondered if his mastectomy had any special meaning for him. "It's strange you should ask that question," she replied. She revealed that John's sister had died one year earlier on November 3 following a mastectomy for breast cancer. Moreover, the wife's sister had died two years earlier on November 12, also from breast cancer following mastectomy. As if this were not momentous enough, John's older and favorite brother had dropped dead of a heart attack one year earlier on November 12. John's death occurred on November 6.

The wife added that she was glad John had not gone further into the garden. Had he done so, he would have discovered that their new trailer had also been spray-painted in black.[1]

Why does despair kill? Cardiologist Bernard Lown and his colleagues at Harvard Medical School have done much to unravel this mystery. These researchers studied 150 patients who had frequent irregularities of the heartbeat involving the left ventricle, the main pumping chamber of the heart. The left ventricle is the part of the heart involved in ventricular fibrillation, the chaotic, ineffective cardiac rhythm that, unless promptly corrected, presages death (this almost certainly was the terminal event in John's case). Of these 150 persons, 117 were followed closely by a team consisting of a psychiatrist and a psychologist in addition to their cardiologists. Of these 117, 62 had one or more episodes of ventricular fibrillation.

The team of specialists discovered that three major factors seemed to be operating in the origin of these life-threatening problems. First, there was the actual *physical disease:* the majority did have atherosclerosis or "hardening" of the coronary arteries. Second, there was the presence of a *psychological state* that was intense enough to pervade and burden daily life. Most frequently either significant depression or a sense of psychological entrapment led to overwhelming despair and helplessness. And third, there was a *psychological trigger event* for the ventricular fibrillation, some happening that was highly meaningful for the person.

John is a classic example of someone with all three factors present. He had had a heart attack; he was enduring a chronic psychological burden, which included fear of losing his job and the accompanying feelings of inadequacy; and, finally, a trigger event— the destruction of his personal property—issued in an avalanche of helplessness and crushing despair. In addition, he faced the anniversaries of the deaths of his sister, brother, and sister-in-law, who died from problems similar to his own, which no doubt added to his sense of futility.

Lown suggests that no single factor out of the three is responsible for ventricular fibrillation; rather, it is the result of a dynamic interplay among all of them. Sometimes the physical factors appear more prominent, sometimes the psychological. If the heart's electrical state is highly unstable, as might be when severe atherosclerosis is present in the coronary arteries, a trivial psychological trigger event may initiate ventricular fibrillation. On the other hand, if little or no underlying heart disease is present, the heart may be relatively immune even to extremely stressful events.[2]

The word "fibrillation" is derived from the Latin *fibrilla,* or "small fiber filament." Fibrillation thus suggests something fragile and tenuous, something easily broken. This image fits because the human heart is profoundly susceptible to the influence of emotions, particularly when it is diseased.

Lown's findings show that if we are to prevent deaths from ventricular fibrillation, we must do more than prevent heart disease itself. It's not enough to focus only on keeping the cholesterol level down, not smoking, controlling blood pressure, exercising regularly, maintaining an ideal body weight, and—if all else fails—calling the heart surgeon to perform a coronary artery bypass operation. A thorough approach must also involve coming to terms with the *meanings* we draw from life and the associated emotions. These constitute the psychological triggers such as the killing despair that John felt. But "the meaning of life" is a diffuse concept, with roots in infancy and perhaps even earlier. How can physicians possibly deal with such a deep-rooted issue when confronted with a patient with heart disease, even if they acknowledge the importance of doing so? This dilemma most commonly prompts physicians to focus on what they *can* treat—high cholesterol levels, obesity, high blood pressure, and so forth. Slowly, however, this situation is changing; there is enormously good news. As we will see later, practical methods are being developed to help heart patients modify the meanings they perceive in their lives, thus changing the injurious emotions that accompany them. Fatal despair such as John's *can* be alleviated. The results can be lifesaving.

Dr. George L. Engel of the University of Rochester School of Medicine has long been a pioneer in the field of mind-body interaction. One of his areas of research is "emotional sudden death." Engel points out that this phenomenon has been described from ancient times to the present:

> The Bible tells us that when Ananias was charged by Peter, "You have not lied to man but to God," he fell down dead; so did Sapphira, his wife, when told that "the feet of them which have buried thy husband are at the door and shall carry thee out" (5 Acts 3:6). Emperor Nerva is said to have died of "a violent excess of anger" against a senator who offended him, as did Valentinian while "reproaching with great passion" the deputies of a German tribe. Pope Innocent IV succumbed suddenly to the "morbid effects of grief on his system" soon after the disastrous overthrow of his army by Manfred, and King Philip V is said to have dropped dead when he realized the Spaniards had been defeated. Chilon of Lacedaemon is alleged to have died from joy while embracing his son who had borne away the prize at the Olympic games. Benjamin Rush claimed that the doorkeeper of Congress, an aged man, died immediately upon hearing the capture of Lord Cornwallis's army. "His death was universally ascribed to a violent emotion of political joy." In more modern times

the power of vengeful deities is no longer invoked, but the belief that intense emotional distress may induce sudden death persists unabated in the average man. Certainly novelists and playwrights have no compunction about arranging for their characters to succumb to a fatal heart attack or stroke in the midst of emotional crisis.[3]

In order to examine the effects of strong emotions on health, Dr. Engel collected, over a six-year period, 170 reports of a sudden death. These came mostly from the Rochester press but also from newspapers of any other cities in which he happened to be. In addition, colleagues learned of his interest and sent him clippings. He used only those reports that had a clear reference to a precipitating life situation, and he excluded all instances where suicide could be even a remote possibility. In 16 cases he was able to get firsthand information from witnesses, the medical examiner, or the hospital involved.

Most of the deaths happened within an hour of the reported emotional event. Of the 170 persons, 99 were males, 64 were females, and 7 persons' gender was not specified. The men were younger on average, with 59 percent being under age sixty-one, compared to only 25 percent of the women. The peak age period for men was approximately fifty, and for women approximately seventy.

The different settings of the sudden deaths and the percentage of deaths that occurred in each were as follows:[4]

SETTING	PERCENTAGE OF DEATHS
1. On the collapse or death of a close person	21%
2. During the period of acute grief (within 16 days)	20%
3. Threat of the loss of a close person	9%
4. During mourning or the anniversary of the death of a close person	3%
5. Loss of status or self-esteem	6%
6. Personal danger or threat of injury, whether real or symbolic	27%

7. After danger is over   7%
8. Reunion, triumph, or "happy end-
   ing"   6%
                                                    ————
                                                     99%

The final two categories may seem troublesome—sudden death after danger has passed and on happy occasions such as reunions and triumphs. These make up 13 percent of the 170 reports. Typical of these accounts, although historical in nature, is the following: "U.S. founding fathers John Adams and Thomas Jefferson . . . both died on the 50th anniversary of the signing of the Declaration of Independence. As recorded by his doctor, Jefferson's last words were, 'Is it the Fourth?' "[5]

Engel's research suggests that both the *intensity* of the emotion and whether it is *negative* or *positive* are important. But rather than conclude that we are all potential victims of positive emotions, we should put these "deaths from happiness" into perspective. We actually know very little about them. In addition to the dramatic trigger event, was there a chronic, burdensome psychological state in the person's life and was underlying heart disease present? It would be a profound mistake to interpret Engel's findings as proof that we should try to walk an emotional tightrope, afraid either to cry or laugh. In fact, it is likely that the media present a seriously exaggerated picture of "deaths from happiness." Just as airline crashes are news, but not the thousands of planes that land safely every day, so, too, are sensational cases in which intensely positive feelings are associated with death, not the many cases in which they are healthy. If we fear that we shall sooner or later become victims of happiness or that we will suddenly be struck dead by a surge of elation, we are drawing the wrong lesson. If we take good care of both our mind and body, eliminating the predisposing factors that set the stage for emotional sudden death, the chances of such an occurrence are utterly remote.

Engel discovered that one of the most frequent settings preceding emotional sudden death is the sense of impasse, where persons believe they can neither fight nor escape. They feel trapped, and they die. The experience of impasse seemed so important that Engel gave it a special name, the "giving up–given up" complex. A typical example is described by J. C. Coolidge, another investigator of these events:

A 45-year-old woman undergoing psychoanalysis . . . had a growing belief that death was the only possible solution for an intolerable situation. She felt a hopeless inability to resolve the problems of an unhappy marriage that she believed would destroy her, and she felt too old and too afraid of being alone to break away to start a life anew. She collapsed an hour after what she interpreted as a rejection by her analyst and within several minutes after a rejection by her husband. This had been preceded by the deaths within 7 months of both parents and a disappointing visit to her only daughter. Rushed to a hospital, she was pulseless and [died] . . . in ventricular fibrillation.[6]

L. J. Saul, a keen observer of the impact of emotions on health, also describes a man whose only outlets for action seemed blocked:

A 45-year-old man found himself in a totally unbearable situation and felt forced to move to another town. But just as he was ready to make the move difficulties developed in the other town that made the move impossible. In an anguished quandary, he, nonetheless, boarded the train for the new locale. Halfway to his destination, he got out to pace the platform at a station stop. When the conductor called, "All aboard," he felt he could neither go on nor return home; he dropped dead on the spot. He was traveling with a friend, a professional person, with whom he shared his awful dilemma. Necropsy showed myocardial infraction [heart attack as the cause of death].[7]

Dr. Joel E. Dimsdale of Harvard Medical School postulates that the following chain of events takes place in emotionally triggered instances of sudden death.[8]

As Figure 1 indicates, it is not just the *presence* of stress that matters in sudden death. Some people, after all, thrive on stress. Something more is involved—the second link in Dimsdale's chain— the *interpretation* of the event by the person. This is how life meanings enter the body, for they *are* our interpretations. Consider once more the case of John's Halloween death. John interpreted the final events of his life in terms of hopelessness, which became the central meaning of his life. He had had a heart attack, was beaten, and there was nothing he could do. This despair and resignation carried over into his response to the final trigger event, the Halloween pranks. His

SETTING FOR EMOTIONAL CAUSES OF SUDDEN DEATH

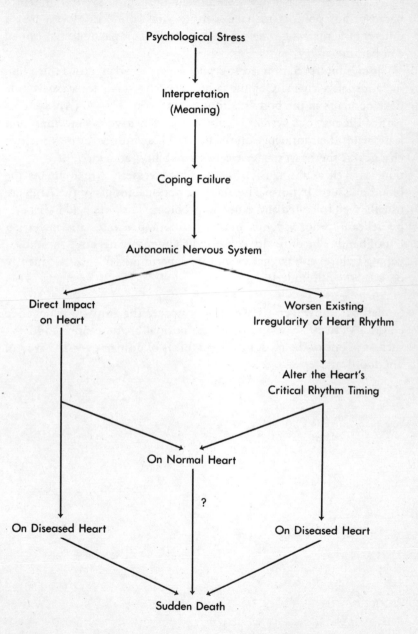

Figure 1.

wife, on the other hand, interpreted the same event differently because she appeared to have a more vital connection with life, a different life meaning. She did not resort to silent passivity but fumed and became angry.

John's interpretation led to *coping failure,* the dangerous third link in Dimsdale's chain. Coping failure sets the stage for catastrophic developments in the body's autonomic nervous system (ANS). This part of the nervous system is enormously sensitive to emotions, and it mediates their influence on the heart. These influences may include changes in the heart's rate, electrical stability, and force of contraction, as well as the tension in the blood vessels, which affects the blood pressure. In normal hearts the emotional inputs of the ANS are usually well tolerated and cause no problem. They are held in balance by delicate feedback loops and homeostatic processes and never get out of hand. The difficulty comes when intensely negative meanings, coping failure, and trigger events are superimposed, most frequently on a heart with underlying disease.

Sometimes, however, as we will now see, the impact of negative emotions can be so severe that even normal hearts cannot endure— such as in one of the most profound forms of despair ever discovered: voodoo death.

Voodoo Death:
The "No Exit" Syndrome

In his classic study of death by voodoo, the great physiologist Walter Cannon relates a case originally recorded by the explorer Mcrolla in his diary during a voyage down the Congo in 1692:

> A young Negro on a journey lodged in a friend's house for the night. The friend had prepared for their breakfast a wild hen, a food strictly banned by a rule which must be inviolably observed. . . . The young fellow demanded whether it was indeed a wild hen and when the host answered "no," he ate it heartily and proceeded on his way. A few years later when the two met again, the old man asked the younger if he would eat a wild hen. He answered that he had been solemnly charged by a wizard not to eat that food. Thereupon the host began to laugh and asked him why he refused it now after having eaten it at his table before. On hearing this news the Negro immediately began to tremble, so greatly was he possessed by fear, and in less than 24 hours he was dead.[1]

"Voodoo cases" illustrate dramatically that—to use the words of writer Norman Cousins—"belief becomes biology."[2] In these cases, the *interpretation* of the event—the significance and meaning it holds for the person—overshadows the event itself, which may be trivial.

The above case shows the *transtemporal* power of meaning, its ability to persist far into the future when the event in question is recalled in the memory. Meaning knows no time; its power can actually *increase* with time. This fact is obvious from "anniversary deaths," in which a person dies on the anniversary of a loved one's death, often many years later.

Cannon, who reported the above case of voodoo, is well known for describing the "fight or flight" concept, in which the body responds to dangers by two different but complementary pathways. He was fascinated by the interplay of mind and body in all its expressions, and wanted to know how charms and spells did their work. He was convinced that the social customs of primitive tribes must somehow play a significant role, for the customs, beliefs, and behaviors determined the significance, interpretation, and meaning of any particular event. Cannon believed that the American psychologist William James had come close to an explanation of voodoo. In his study, Cannon cited this passage from James's *Principles of Psychology:*

> A man's social me is the recognition which he gets from his mates. We are not only gregarious animals, liking to be in sight of our fellows, but we have an innate propensity to get ourselves noticed, and noticed favorably, by our kind. No more fiendish punishment could be devised, were such a thing physically possible, than that one should be turned loose in society and remain absolutely unnoticed by all the members thereof. If no one turned round when we entered, answered when we spoke, or minded what we did, but if every person we met "cut us dead," or acted as if we were non-existing things, a kind of rage and impotent despair would ere long well up in us, from which the cruelest bodily tortures would be a relief; for these would make us feel that, however bad might be our plight, we had not sunk to such a depth as to be unworthy of attention at all.[3]

Cannon discovered that cultures practicing voodoo had various ways of bringing "malignant psychic influences" to bear on the victim, *all* of which depended on the impact of perceived meaning. For example, the person might be hexed by having a special bone pointed at him, by being stuck with a "poisoned" spear that was actually harmless, or by unknowingly eating a forbidden food. The primary factor in all these instances seemed to be the meaning the event contained for the person against whom it was directed. But this is only half the process. Not only does the meaning sink into the mind of the victim, it spreads through the supporting social group as well. Cannon described this dynamic and the macabre results that followed:

> There are two definite movements . . . in the process by which black magic becomes effective on the victim. . . . In the first movement the community contracts [away from him] . . . and places him in a new category. He is now viewed as one who is more nearly in the realm of the sacred and tabu than in the world of the ordinary where the community finds itself. . . . He is alone and isolated. . . . The only escape is by death. During the death illness which ensues, the group acts . . . with countless stimuli to suggest death positively to the victim, who is in a highly suggestible state. In addition . . . the victim . . . as a rule, not only makes no effort to live . . . but actually . . . coöperates in the withdrawal. . . . He becomes what the attitude of his fellow tribesmen will him to be. Thus he assists in committing a kind of suicide.
>
> Before death takes place, the second movement of the community occurs, which is a return to the victim in order to subject him to the fateful ritual of mourning. . . . [This] place[s] him in . . . the sacred totemic world of the dead.
> The effect . . . is obviously drastic.[4]

An understatement, to say the least.

Even in voodoo there is room for hope, and the outcome is not always fatal. The impending tragedy can be aborted by the medicine man. He knows that meanings for the victim and the tribe are not fixed but malleable, and he is a master at creating new meaning—usually by counteracting the spell with the power of the countercharm.[5]

MODERN-DAY VOODOO

We should not smugly assume that voodoo death is limited to "primitives" and that we have risen above them on this score. Modern societies are not yet finished with death curses; we allow them to slip into our cultural life in subtle ways. At times we manifest precisely the same double movements Cannon so clearly described.[6]

An example is the way we deal with the elderly, who are effectively cursed by the act of growing old and feeble in a society that fanatically values youthfulness and vigor. We behave differently toward the elderly and they know it. Like the person under a voodoo curse, they often cooperate by behaving like an "old person." When they are consigned to a nursing home or a retirement village they may offer momentary objections at being shut off from the social group, but they usually comply with the will of the family and the expectations of the society as a whole. This "spell" is intensified on entering the nursing home and being surrounded by others under the same curse, who have come to the same place to live out their role as old persons in accordance with the expectations of their own families. Social support and visitation is all too often gradually withdrawn by families: the old person, like the voodoo victim, ceases to exist. As James and Cannon clearly saw, frequently the only recourse in such a situation is death, in which the old person obligingly cooperates with his curse.

A second example of "the curse" in action in modern society is in the events surrounding the diagnosis of malignant disease. Even though the physician dutifully describes the prognosis and the "survival" statistics, the curse frequently has already done its work. Even though patients may be told they have a 50 percent chance of living another five years, their interpretation is frequently that they have a 50 percent chance of dying. Like the accursed individual in voodoo societies, they may cooperate by succumbing "on time."

A third example is forced retirement. For many people, especially men, the sense of identity, dignity, significance, and self-worth is tightly bound to their work. When work is taken away, they no longer feel real—the predeath psychological state in voodoo societies. Death statistics reveal the effects: forced retirement, mainly in men, resembles a death sentence.

The antidote for modern-day voodoo is the same as in primitive voodoo: the restoration of meaning for the accursed. For example, psychologists Ellen Langer and Judith Rodin "changed the meaning" of the nursing home experience for a group of elderly patients by giving them control and responsibility. These patients were given potted plants to care for and were offered suggestions on doing more for themselves, such as planning their own menus, instead of letting the staff take all the responsibility. A second group, similar to the first in terms of health problems and disabilities, received the usual approach. They were told the staff would be responsible for all aspects of their care and would make all the decisions. Within only three weeks the first group demonstrated significant improvements in their health and their level of physical activity. These results were even more dramatic after eighteen months. Restoration of meaning appeared genuinely lifesaving: at the end of the eighteen-month study, the death rate of the "self-responsibility" group was only one-half that of the other.[7]

One of the commonest forms of despair, "no exit," or impasse is the feeling of being trapped in a job one does not like. The effects of job dissatisfaction are so profound they have been given a special name: Black Monday syndrome.

Black Monday Syndrome:

When Dread Means Dead

After I came home from the hospital to recover from my heart attack, I was sitting in my backyard watching the birds flitting and chattering. It was Monday. Ordinarily I would have been very unhappy on Monday— the first day of the week back at the office with the whole week ahead of me. But the birds didn't know it was Monday; they're just as happy on Monday as on Friday. Suddenly I wondered if the dread I have of Mondays had something to do with my health. I had my heart attack on Monday.

My patient was sitting in my office as he chatted, having come for his first checkup after being discharged from the hospital. Although he had experienced a stormy course after his heart attack, he was now doing well. All on his own, he had stumbled onto a tantalizing fact while watching the birds in his backyard: *More fatal heart attacks occur on Monday than on any other day of the week.*[1]

This is extraordinarily bizarre. As far as we know, *no other living creature* manages to die more frequently on a particular day of the week.

How could our heart know which *day* it is? Presumably the cholesterol deposits that may be clogging its arteries are just as unaware of the day of the week as the birds my patient was observing. If heart attacks are due only to "physical" reasons, why should Black Monday syndrome exist?

To be sure, physical reasons have been proposed to explain Black Monday syndrome. Perhaps some persons are reexposed to job-related chemicals on Monday, after being free of them on the weekend, the reexposure triggering some untoward event much like an allergic reaction. Or perhaps the overeating and drinking that are more common on the weekend somehow play a role. But so far none of these physical possibilities have been proved.

Could the *meaning* of Monday be the difference? Could it be that human beings, creatures who are uniquely sensitive to the meanings in life, are paying a terrible price on returning to jobs and work situations they despise? This possibility is supported by the fact that heart attacks not only are more frequent on Mondays, but *cluster around 9:00 A.M.*—the very hour on which the new workweek begins.

The health risk of being chronically unhappy in a job has been known for some time. In 1972 a study done in Massachusetts for the Department of Health, Education and Welfare found that the best predictor for heart disease was *not* any of the major *physical* risk factors (smoking, high blood pressure, elevated cholesterol, and diabetes mellitus) but *job dissatisfaction*. And the second best predictor was what the researchers called "overall happiness."[2] This finding fits with the fact that most persons below the age of fifty in this country who have their first heart attack have *none* of the major physical risk factors for coronary artery disease.[3] These findings suggest that in our understanding of coronary artery disease, which kills more people in our society than all other diseases combined, something vitally important has been left out.

A "solution" to Black Monday syndrome was offered by another heart attack patient of mine. During his recovery phase we discussed his intense dislike of his job. The next week he returned to announce triumphantly, "I've got the answer! I'm skipping Mondays! I'm going to return to work on Tuesday!" He missed the point. There is nothing malevolent about Monday. It is the day of the return that seems to matter, not the particular day on which the return falls. If the workweek began on Tuesday, we would probably be referring to Black Tuesday syndrome.

The researcher who has done most to bring these Monday

morning findings to light is Dr. James E. Muller of Harvard Medical School.[4] In the spring of 1984 when he was lecturing on heart disease, someone from the audience commented that his data suggested that more heart attacks occur in winter than in summer. That sounded reasonable to Muller because it fit the stereotype of a middle-aged man shoveling snow and clutching his chest with a heart attack. But when he examined his data further, the correlation with winter could not be substantiated; heart attacks were equally distributed throughout the year. Instead, Muller found something more surprising— heart attacks tended to occur around 9:00 A.M. Initially he thought this was a spurious finding: "I thought it was an artifact," he remembers. But when he began looking for confirmation he found fourteen studies, all published "in obscure journals," suggesting the same thing.

"Once I found those studies, I began to believe the finding was real, and I reasoned that if heart attacks are caused by blood clots that occur in the morning, perhaps strokes are too," he says. His reasoning was that strokes, our third leading cause of death, are also a disease of the cardiovascular system and might show a similar variation. To test this possibility, Muller contacted experts at the National Institutes of Health, where there is a data bank on over 1,000 stroke patients. He found that no one had ever looked for a time when strokes occur. A computer search was begun, and it quickly became obvious that the stroke data were even stronger than the heart attack data: strokes occur most commonly between 8:00 and 9:00 A.M. The incidence of strokes is lowest between 3:00 and 4:00 A.M.

What about sudden deaths in general? Might they also show the same variation? Dr. Paul Ludmer, who had worked with Muller, examined the time of death on death certificates of all persons who died suddenly in Massachusetts in 1983. There were twice as many sudden deaths at 9:00 A.M. as at 5:00 A.M., when the incidence was lowest.

Currently the attempts to unravel these curious findings are focused on a biochemical explanation. Investigators are looking at those circadian rhythms (bodily processes that vary within a twenty-four hour period) that change in the early morning hours and might trigger heart attack and stroke. There are several candidates. It is known that heart rate and blood pressure rise in the early morning hours. There are also circadian rhythms involving the stickiness of the platelets in the blood, which might make clots in the coronary or cerebral arteries more likely. Surges in chemicals such as adrenaline also occur in the morning, and these increases might stimulate the coronary arteries to contract, predisposing to heart attack.

Although these circadian changes might explain why, in general, heart attacks and strokes are more prominent at a particular time of *day*, they do not help us understand why they cluster on a certain day of the *week*. And even though circadian rhythms may be important, this does not rule out a coexistent role for emotions. Emotions can trigger biochemical changes of their own, which might act in concert with circadian flows. Studies of subordinate primates—for example, male baboons forced by dominant males into inferior roles—show that chronically stressed animals indeed have higher elevations of certain stress hormones that can have negative effects on heart function. Platelet aggregation or stickiness also is known to increase in persons under psychological stress, which might be more pronounced on Monday in someone returning to a job they dread.

What are the practical implications of these findings? Dr. Michael Rocco of Harvard Medical School suggests ways of counteracting the biochemical events before they have a chance to harm the heart. For example, heart patients could take quick-acting drugs when they awaken in the morning or longer-acting medications on going to bed at night. But if the "meaning of Monday" is important in the genesis of these problems—if the emotional responses of the person play a role—then factors such as job satisfaction and "overall happiness" also need to be dealt with.[5]

Job satisfaction seems to play a crucial role in other health problems as well. A recent study examined the incidence of low back pain in 31,200 employees at the Boeing Company in the Seattle–Tacoma area. Surprisingly, there was no difference in incidence of low back pain and disability between white- and blue-collar workers. It did not seem to matter whether the employee stood on an assembly line or sat at a desk. The best explanatory factor was job satisfaction, which had been assessed by job ratings by supervisors within the six months prior to the back problem.[6]

There is also evidence that some workers have a higher-than-average risk of heart attack—for example, waiters, gasoline station attendants, and certain data processors. In these jobs, the worker is powerless to control the work load. No matter how high the volume, one can only struggle harder to cope with it. If the work load is excessive and protracted, the situation begins to resemble the "learned helplessness" situation described by researchers in animal behavior.

It is not difficult to understand how any employee could develop an indwelling sense of entrapment and helplessness in a similar situation, especially if controlled by supervisors who are insensitive to these issues. But this does *not* mean that anyone working in any particular occupation is doomed to a heart attack. After all, *most* busy waiters, gas station attendants, and data processors *don't* experience myocardial infarctions. These are statistical findings only; while they indicate an increase in the *risk* for a heart attack they certainly do not guarantee one. And in any case, most jobs *can* be structured in ways that give the employee an element of control, preventing a feeling of resignation and impasse—and hopefully neutralizing the effects of Black Monday.

THE CURE FOR BLACK MONDAY: THE 3 Cs

Not only do most people in stressful jobs not succumb to Black Monday syndrome, many of them *never get sick*. Over the past decade psychologists have studied these resilient, hardy people. As a result, many researchers have concluded that it is not job stress that is most important in determining health or illness, but rather, *how we respond to it*. This means there is an antidote to Black Monday syndrome, a way to avoid its effects.

A team of behavioral scientists at the University of Chicago, led by psychologists Suzanne Kobasa and Salvatore Maddi, studied a group of 200 business executives at Illinois Bell Telephone Company who were subjected to enormous stresses during the AT&T divestiture.[7] Even before the divestiture, stress was a factor: so many executives had experienced heart attacks by age fifty that the company actually had installed a cardiac unit in its corporate headquarters! Half of the executives in the study reported numerous symptoms and health problems, and half did not. Yet they were subjected to the same job stress. What made the difference? Kobasa and her colleagues found major psychological differences in the two groups. Those who stayed healthy judged their stresses differently and responded to them differently than the illness-prone group. The healthy individuals possessed what the psychologists called a capacity for "optimistic cognitive appraisal," meaning that they had a way of "seeing the cup half-full rather than half-empty." When stressful events occurred, they did not regard them as the end of the world but as a natural and inevitable part of their lives. This allowed their bodies to respond to stress differently, averting injurious biochemical responses. In effect these people could *control* their body's reaction to stress. They also interpreted stress differently by regarding it as a *challenge,* an opportunity to learn, grow, and become a wiser, better manager. Not only were the healthy executives deeply involved in their work, they had a strong *commitment* to their families and to life in general off the job. Kobasa and her team thus identified the "3 Cs"—control, challenge, and commitment—as the key factors behind the hardy personality that remains healthy under stress.

How can we acquire a sense of control in a job involving situations that are clearly beyond our power to change? As psychologist Blair Justice points out, *the sense of control is largely a belief.*[8] It does *not* mean having an iron grip on all the people and circumstances around us so that we can manipulate or force them into complying with all our wishes. This type of control reflects the need for power and, as research has shown, is not health promoting but actually destructive to health.[9] Moreover, difficult, sometimes uncontrollable circumstances are a fact of life off the job as well as on the job. Yet studies have shown that even under the worst circumstances we can imagine, such as war, torture, or concentration camps, people *can* retain a sense of control and remain healthy. In fact, some people in these dire situations become *healthier* than previously if their sense of control remains intact.[10]

In situations we cannot change, the sense of control seems largely to flow from an inner certainty or faith about one's place or role in life. Sociologist Aaron Antonovsky calls this a "sense of coherence,"[11] and researcher Thomas Boyce terms it a "sense of permanence and continuity."[12] Belief in a supreme being facilitates this awareness for some people.

The sense of control in difficult circumstances correlates also with ego strength. A sense of self-esteem, individual worthiness, dignity, and integrity help make up a healthy ego. These perceptions about "who we are" make it possible for us to appraise optimistically the harsh realities of life, engage them, and change them whenever possible.

As our awareness of the negative effects of stress has increased, it is possible that we have overemphasized the role of the stress itself and undervalued the protective, healing power within ourselves. We should always recall that, no matter how stressful the event, we can always bring our attitudes, beliefs, and meanings to bear on the situation and change its effects on us—even Black Monday.

In addition to an unsatisfactory job situation, there are many other ways people can feel trapped in our society and lose all sense of control. One of the most devastating is being illiterate and poorly educated. As we shall now see, there is evidence that illiteracy and the feelings of isolation that go with it are highly toxic to the heart.

Johnny Can't Read, Johnny Has Heart Disease:
Education, Isolation, and Health

> [Poor education is] an Orwellian recipe in which the estranged worker, besieged from above and below, mixes internal rage and incessant frustration into a fatal brew.
>
> —THOMAS B. GRABOYS,
> Harvard Medical School[1]

In the 1989 movie *Stanley and Iris,* Stanley, played by actor Robert De Niro, is illiterate. Although he is brilliant and is a closet inventor, he is employed as a humble cafeteria worker in a factory.

His job makes few demands and he is good at it, but his illiteracy is his undoing. Although Stanley's boss admits Stanley is a good worker, he becomes worried that Stanley might "hurt somebody" as a result of his handicap and fires him. Stanley rides a bicycle everywhere because he cannot pass a driver's test, read street signs, or identify bus routes. Cut off from normal relationships by his profound disability, he lives, in a quiet rage, with his aging father.

One day a simple event almost pushes him over the edge. He stops at a shoe repair shop to pick up his shoes, but the cobbler won't release them unless he signs for them. Rules are rules: no signature, no shoes. Stanley is trapped—a genuine impasse, a "no exit" situation. Like a cornered animal, he becomes enraged. He suddenly leaps the counter, menaces the employee, grabs the shoes, and storms out of the shop.

The triviality of the event is telling: in the life of almost anyone, picking up an item at a shoe repair shop is an experience of little consequence. But the illiterate person lives with a constant, daily dread of these simple experiences because they can escalate to become monumental challenges and an affront to personal dignity.

Each day of Stanley's life is oriented toward disguising his disability and "faking it." The resulting pathos and aloneness are immense. Stanley eventually falls in love with Iris, a factory worker with enormous compassion and patience. She teaches him to read and write, and finally he escapes the prison of illiteracy.

Stanley's story ends in triumph; it is, after all, a movie. But for many illiterates there are no happy endings. In fact, there is increasing evidence that illiteracy and the emotions that accompany it are some of the most toxic forms of life experience we know.

In 1984, Dr. William Ruberman and his colleagues interviewed 2,320 male survivors of heart attacks. After controlling for the influence of well-known factors such as cigarette smoking, blood pressure, cholesterol, diabetes, and many others, Ruberman's team found that those patients who were socially isolated and who had a high degree of life stress had *more than four times* the risk of death than men with low levels of isolation and stress. Moreover, the *poorly educated* had the most social isolation and life stress, and the best-educated had the least. In fact, the poorly educated had the highest risk of dying.[2]

Why do poorly educated persons have poorer health? Some people think they simply take worse care of themselves: they smoke more, exercise less, eat unwisely, and have less access to good health care. But it is possible to take these factors into account by using sophisticated methods of analysis, and to determine their relative impact on health. Thus Ruberman's team was able to show that smoking, exercise, diet, and accessibility to health care, while important, did not explain the poorer health and earlier death of these persons; the influence of social isolation and poor education was more powerful.

But which was more important—social isolation and stress or low education levels? Again the researchers were able to tease apart these factors by standard methods. They concluded that poor education was only a stand-in or "proxy" for stress and loneliness—that is, low education actually did its damage through the stress and social isolation to which it led.

In another well-known study, done in Alameda County, California, approximately 7,000 people were surveyed about their level of social interaction. Their contacts with friends and relatives, church membership, marital status, and many other indicators of social connectedness were tabulated in detail. The survey took into consideration not only the number but the intensity of relationships. Nine years later the mortality level of the group was assessed. For all ages and both sexes, mortality was greatest for those with the lowest degree of social interaction. Death rates were highest among the true loners, those with the fewest relationships. This correlation remained significant even when factors such as socioeconomic status, cigarette smoking, and other health practice variables were considered and removed. Isolation was correlated with higher death rates from coronary artery disease, cancer, and all other major diagnoses including suicide and accidental death. But the chicken-or-the-egg question arises: did loneliness and isolation cause the various diseases or did the diseases cause the loneliness and isolation? The researchers found that the causal factors were loneliness and isolation.[3] Another well-known study, done in Tecumseh, Michigan, confirmed that increased loneliness and absence of social networks were the cause and not the result of disease and illness.[4]

What does "being lonely" mean? As epidemiologist Leonard A. Sagan states in his important book The Health of Nations, loneliness is quite different from merely being alone. Many people actually benefit from periods of isolation; being alone can be restorative and can provide an opportunity for contemplation and reflection. On the other hand, there are persons who feel isolated and lonely even in groups or crowds. So it's not just the number of persons with whom we surround ourselves that counts. Something more is involved, which is apparently the *perception* of isolation and the actual *satisfaction* that our relationships bring.[5]

How is poor education related to isolation and loneliness? "Reading and writing are more than technical skills or tools," Sagan states. "The ability to communicate provides an opportunity to be sensitive to one's own feelings, to communicate and relate with others in a meaningful way, to achieve a sense of competence that the illiterate can rarely gain."[6] Sagan's message: the inability to read and write sets one apart; being illiterate means being alone.

How do social isolation and poor social status actually cause the physical changes of poor health and earlier death? Studies of primates have yielded many clues. For instance, in groups of baboons living in the wild, life for low-ranking, low-status animals is often miserable. It consists of hard-earned, stolen meals and harassment by dominant males that can be life-threatening. The low-ranking male, even if he never picks a fight, is in constant danger of being assaulted and must always be on guard. In short, his entire life is spent with little control. These social stresses correlate with pathological biochemical changes internally. Subordinate baboon males have the type of physiology found in stress-related diseases. Their blood level of hydrocortisone, a hormone secreted during stress, is high and remains elevated even after a stressful event is over. Low-ranking males have lower concentrations of high-density lipoproteins (HDL), which are known to carry the "good" type of cholesterol and protect against heart disease. They have weaker immune systems, with fewer circulating lymphocytes to detect invading pathogens. And during stress they cannot maintain adequate levels of testosterone, the sex hormone that is valuable for muscle metabolism and aggression.[7]

This scenario is similar to the experience of poorly educated or illiterate persons: they, too, spend their lives on the margins of society looking on, unable to compete effectively. They have little autonomy or control over what happens to them, which often leads to a chronic and debilitating sense of despair, futility, and anger. They frequently exert enormous effort to disguise their handicap, all the while knowing they are living a lie. This strategy usually fails, and a chronic sense of isolation becomes a way of life. When an illiterate person *resigns* himself or herself to never learning to read and write, an authentic "no exit" or impasse situation is in place.

In spite of excellent studies such as those above, the problems of illiteracy and loneliness still largely go unrecognized by physicians, health care planners, and politicians, who prefer to attack illness on the other end: devising treatments *after* diseases have occurred rather than before. Social isolation and poor education are generally considered outside the medical arena altogether. By and large, doing diagnostic studies and using drugs and surgery are considered by physicians to be glamorous and interesting; inquiring about literacy and relationships is not.

The above studies suggest, however, that we will never solve the problem of heart disease by focusing only on physical factors—cholesterol, blood pressure, smoking, diabetes, diet, exercise, and so forth. Although important, these risk factors give an incomplete picture of our number one killer. As we have already observed, most persons in the United States who have their first heart attack below the age of fifty have *none* of the "big four" major risk factors present.[8] Unless we also devote attention to the neglected twin factors of educational levels and social isolation, winning the "war on heart disease" will be like fighting with one hand tied behind our back.

If one is admitted to the hospital for heart disease or other illness, what then? We will see that another set of problems then surface, problems that can only be understood, once again, by taking meanings and emotions into account.

EIGHT

The Patient Patient:
The Hazards of the Medical Experience

What does it mean to be a patient?

"Being patient" means having endurance, forbearance, persever-ance, and the ability to wait passively without complaining. All these qualities go into being a patient. Our words "pathos" and "passion" also are related to the word "patient" in the original Latin meaning, and in times past "patient" referred to suffering, agony, and intense emotion.

Today, being a patient suggests having an uncomplaining attitude, doing as we're told, silently submitting to whatever a health care expert tells us is good for us—basically assuming a position of helplessness. But as many "good" patients who adopt this attitude discover, the old meanings are not dead. As these patients become increasingly helpless, they feel the original meaning of "patient" surface; intense emotion and suffering bubble up, and some of them even die.

At the same time the "good" patient is being passive, another process is taking place in the body—the innate drive in higher organisms to *act* or *do* something when threatened, to either fight back or flee the dangerous situation. This urge creates a dilemma because the "good" or "patient" patient cannot allow himself or herself to do this. Thus he or she experiences an emotional double bind because both options—doing nothing and taking action—seem un-acceptable. The result is often a feeling of utter despair and helpless-ness—the "no exit" or impasse which, as we have seen, can be fatal.

As the following two cases show, a sense of despair and entrapment can arise even from simple, everyday medical experiences, such as being stuck with a needle:

A 44-year-old woman with no particular complaints was scheduled for a routine venipuncture as part of a general checkup. Because the patient was always extremely fearful about having blood drawn, and usually fainted, the precaution was taken of placing her in a recumbent position. Within seconds of the needle's puncturing the vein, she complained of feeling weak, broke out into a cold sweat, turned pale, and went into cardiac arrest. No heart sounds were audible, carotid and femoral pulses were absent, there was no spontaneous breathing, and her pupils became widely dilated. Immediate cardiopulmonary resuscitation was instituted, and the patient regained consciousness approximately 2 min[utes] later. Recovery was complete within 15 min[utes]. She refused hospitalization and left the office on her own power. When seen 18 months later she had remained well. [1]

A 55-year-old man, who had had his first myocardial infarction 6 months earlier, was being worked up in the emergency department for what proved to be a second infarction, when he developed ventricular fibrillation and cardiac arrest. He was promptly and successfully resuscitated. Interviewed several days later, the patient reported that he had been feeling pain-free and relatively comfortable until the house officer began what proved to be an unsuccessful effort to do an arterial puncture. As the intern persevered in his fruitless endeavor, the patient became apprehensive, concerned about the doctor's competence, and then overwhelmed with a sense of impotence to do anything about his situation. During these several minutes he first felt hot and flushed, his chest pain returned, and then while the intern was out of the room looking for someone to help him with the arterial puncture, the patient became weak and then suddenly passed out. [2]

Many patients trust their physician implicitly and are prepared to believe anything he or she says. For them the doctor's utterances may have oracular power. Many sensitive physicians realize the power of their words and use them purposefully to bring about healing effects in their patients. Some, however, do not. When a patient hangs on the physician's every word, and when the physician is insensitive to their effects, a potentially lethal brew forms.

An example is related by Jon Kabat-Zinn, who developed and heads the Stress Reduction Clinic of the University of Massachusetts Medical School. This case history is adapted from his excellent book *Full Catastrophe Living:*

Dr. Bernard Lown, the noted Harvard cardiologist, was completing his training some thirty years ago at Harvard Medical School under the tutelage of the noted heart specialist Dr. S. A. Levine. Dr. Levine was a consummate clinician who possessed an awesome presence, and it is said that his patients hung on his every word. He was noted for being invariably reassuring, caring, and convincing to those he served.

On one occasion in the cardiac clinic the trainees were examining a patient, waiting for Dr. Levine to drop in to discuss their findings and review the case. The patient, Mrs. S., was well known to Dr. Levine, having been followed in the heart clinic for a decade. A middle-aged librarian, she had a narrowing of the tricuspid valve on the right side of the heart, and experienced low-grade, chronic congestive heart failure. However, with the help of medications, she maintained her job and attended to her household chores.

Dr. Levine entered the examining room, greeted Mrs. S. warmly, examined her, and then turned to the large entourage of trainees and said, "This woman has TS," and abruptly left. No sooner had he exited than Mrs. S.'s demeanor changed abruptly. She appeared fearful and began to breathe rapidly and deeply, obviously hyperventilating. Soon her skin was drenched with perspiration, and her pulse increased to more than 150 per minute. On reexamining her, Dr. Lown found that her lungs were filling with fluid, although they were clear a few minutes earlier. This was remarkable, because the right-sided heart valve problem usually caused no accumulation of fluid in the lungs.

Dr. Lown asked her why she was so upset. She replied that Dr. Levine had said that she had TS, which she knew meant "terminal situation." This amused Dr. Lown initially, for he knew the acronym stood for "tricuspid stenosis," the condition of her heart valve. Mrs. S. failed, however, to be reassured by this explanation, and her congestion worsened. Her lungs continued to fill with fluid, and she lost consciousness, unable to breathe. Heroic measures did not help. Dr. Lown tried to reach Dr. Levine to see if his further words or presence might make a difference, but he could not be located. Later in the day Mrs. S. died from intractable heart failure.[3]

The following example involves a medical test that is commonplace today, cardiac catheterization. In it, a thin, hollow tube is threaded up a major blood vessel into the heart and the coronary arteries, dye is injected, and X rays are taken. Thousands of persons a year safely undergo cardiac catheterizations; it is regarded as a routine study with minimal risk.

A robust, middle-aged male was to undergo a cardiac catheterization as part of his evaluation for the cause of chest pain. He confessed to his cardiologist prior to the test that he felt his heart would stop during the procedure and that he would die. This revelation was made with considerable embarrassment because he took great pride in his masculinity and his ability to "take anything." The cardiologist assured him that everything would be fine and that his fear of death was for naught. However, during the procedure, which revealed relatively normal coronary arteries, the patient's heartbeat began to gradually slow from 90 beats per minute to the 50s and 40s, and then completely stopped. The man became unconscious and his electrocardiogram revealed a "straight line." Resuscitation procedures were immediately instituted, with complete and uneventful recovery. When interviewed later, he had no recall of the event, stating only that he "knew it would happen."[4]

Rationality and intellectual knowledge are not enough to protect one from the curse of careless words. Even physicians who know all about diagnostic tests can be victims, as shown in the following case of a doctor who underwent a cardiac catheterization:

An anxious, forty-year-old physician sought medical advice for chest pain from a cardiologist, a friend in whom he had great trust. The evaluation led eventually to a cardiac catheterization, which the physician-patient was loath to have because of his fear that something would go wrong. During the test, he was extremely apprehensive. Nonetheless, the test proceeded uneventfully—until the cardiologist carelessly dropped a syringe immediately following the injection of dye into a coronary artery and loudly exclaimed, "Oh, God!" This created profound alarm in the patient, who thought a catastrophe had occurred. He cried, "What happened!" and clutched his chest in severe pain. At the same moment the cardiologist observed on the fluoroscope the cause of the pain: a coronary artery was going into spasm, shutting off blood supply to part of the heart. The patient's hands blanched completely white, as their arteries also went into spasm. This was the first time the patient had ever experienced such an event. Immediate measures were taken, and the blood vessel spasms were relieved. The man recovered without incident. His coronary arteries proved to be normal, free of any obstructions.[5]

These examples show that the hazards of being a patient are not entirely physical in origin, but are based on the meaning and significance the experience has for the person and on his or her interpretation of the situation. Dr. Anthony Lalli of the Cleveland Clinic proposes that the emotions patients experience during invasive X-ray tests may account for *all* the known causes of death associated with these tests. Dr. Lalli studied 248 fatalities that occurred as a result of the use of contrast media, the chemicals injected intravenously to obtain X rays of various organs (kidneys, bladder, liver, lungs, heart, brain, etc.). He examined all the causes of death, including heart attack, ventricular fibrillation, respiratory arrest, pulmonary and cerebral edema, rapid clotting of the blood, inability of the blood to clot normally, and various other causes. He was searching for a unifying explanation that might account for all these different types of fatalities. His conclusion was this: "the most important factors in the production of contrast media reactions are the patient's fear and apprehension."[6]

Lalli does not deny that the chemical that is injected is involved. But the chemical is always used against an emotional backdrop, which all too often includes anxiety, fear, even terror.

These emotions are understandable. The person is usually strapped down and commanded to be immobile during the procedure—the "lie there and take it" position. "Don't breathe, don't talk" are common commands given during the test. Although the fear may mount, the patient realizes that, as we noted above, the usual responses to threat—fight and flight—are impossible. The ensuing sense of "no exit" or impasse can be fed by numerous sensations during the test that convince the person that something is wrong. For instance, he or she may experience a slight feeling of warmth or burning in the arm where the contrast media was injected, or total-body flushing or heat. Of themselves, these events are quite harmless and are extremely common. But for some persons they increase the feeling of entrapment: "Something terrible is happening and there's nothing I can do about it!"

Lalli describes how these emotions affect the brain:

> The brain is primed by the patient's fear or anxiety and the limbic lobe of the cerebrum acts upon the hypothalamus which is awesomely plenipotential in its abilities to produce untoward responses. Through the connections of the hypothalamus with the respiratory center immediate respiratory arrest can occur. The connections with the vasomotor center may plunge the patient directly into shock.[7]

In brief, Lalli's proposal rests on biological facts. The parts of the brain where thought and emotion take place are connected with other brain centers which, in turn, control critical bodily functions such as heartbeat, breathing rate, and blood pressure. Because of these connections, fear and anxiety have a route into most of the organs of the body.

In Part III, "Healing Breakthroughs," we will examine ways persons can change the disturbing emotions that can accompany "patient behavior." One recommendation, however, should be directed to physicians, not patients: Never underestimate the power of words not only to heal but to kill. This warning forms the basis of Lalli's advice to doctors performing invasive X ray tests:

> I would recommend that [physicians] injecting [contrast] materials adopt the mien of equanimity urged upon us by Sir William Osler [the father of American medicine], treat their patients with gentleness and inapparent concern and not arouse their anxieties or increase their fear. . . . The physician–patient dialogue should not center on possible reactions but might best be devoted to the weather.[8]

If hospitals can be hazardous to patients, so can medical schools to medical students. As we shall now see, these effects on medical students, though often immediate, can also be delayed. And sometimes they can even be fatal.

Getting Ahead and Getting Cancer:
The Problems of Being a Medical Student

Medical school would be O.K. if it weren't for the goddamned students.

—COMMENT BY A FAMOUS MEDICAL SCHOOL
FACULTY MEMBER TO A GROUP
OF MEDICAL STUDENTS

In the OR [operating room] I was being taught to suture. When I held the forceps improperly I was hit on the knuckles with another instrument by my chief. When I inadvertently did it again I was hit in the same place. After the operation, my knuckles were bleeding and I now have a scar on the back of my right hand.

—MEDICAL STUDENT[1]

This [abuse] was not so much one major event as repeated ones; daily insults, rude remarks, etc., which went on for the entire 6 weeks [of surgery instruction] and had a significant detrimental effect on my self-confidence for some time afterward. . . . I was told I was worthless. . . . When I did answer correctly, I was never praised but was told the stupidest of medical students should, after all, know this information. . . . I was the only woman on the surgical team, and often rude remarks were made about women in my presence. . . . Occasionally, these were personally directed. The incident which made me angriest (and I do not anger easily) was when, at the conclusion of afternoon rounds, the chief resident stated that I could now come and 'service' him and the third-year resident in the call room. This was not said in a flirtatious manner; it was very derisive in tone. It was obviously meant to anger me, and it did.

—MEDICAL STUDENT[2]

I was examining another student in an ophthalmology practicum, who turned out to have a corneal abrasion from previous tonometry [a measurement of the internal pressure in the eye]. As my classmate was in obvious pain, I wanted to stop the examination. When I explained this to the supervising physician he said, "Oh good, this gives us an opportunity to learn how to force a patient to cooperate even if they are in pain."

—MEDICAL STUDENT[3]

[In the survey] twelve students (16%) had been subjected to actual physical harm. . . . Examples . . . included being slapped, kicked, hit, or having things thrown at them. One student reported he had been kicked in the testicular region by an attending physician and required medical attention for his injury.[4]

Medicine men aren't horses. You don't breed them.

—LAME DEER
Sioux medicine man[5]

One of the hospitals at which I trained was Parkland Memorial Hospital In Dallas, which perhaps is best known as the hospital where President John F. Kennedy was taken when he was shot. I revered the institution as one of the finest teaching hospitals in the country, but I could never understand why young physicians were treated the way they were.

In the early seventies protest was in the air. It was not only women, gays, and blacks who sought change; young doctors and medical students also were irate. Many of the nation's teaching hospitals, including Parkland, became the scene of protests. For us young physicians the key issues were the long hours and low pay. We were earning poverty wages—at one point, I calculated, an average of forty cents an hour for 80 to 100 hours of work a week.

A group of my colleagues decided to confront the administrator of Parkland Hospital with our grievances. A major complaint was the tremendous imbalance between our salaries and the relatively high salaries paid the trainees in hospital administration.

The administrator, well known for his antipathy toward interns and residents, listened impassively. Finally he said simply, "Gentlemen, you don't understand. These hospital administration trainees are *college graduates!*"

The young doctors were stunned. What were *they*? Lower forms of life? Like the hospital administration trainees, they were college graduates and many had advanced degrees as well. In addition they had completed four years of medical school, obtained the M.D. degree, finished a year of internship, and were involved in even more years of fellowship and specialty training. Nothing they said proved convincing, however, and the administrator angrily and abruptly closed the meeting. It was several years before the physicians' complaints began to be redressed.

I forgot about these events until 1976, when I was a private practitioner of internal medicine in Dallas. That year a landmark study was published which vividly stirred my memories of what it is like to be a medical student.

The research dealt with the effects of emotions on health and was done by Dr. Caroline B. Thomas. For almost thirty years she performed psychological tests on every incoming medical student at the Johns Hopkins School of Medicine in Baltimore, Maryland. She followed the students over time, and at the end of the study examined the test scores for correlations between the psychological profiles and the diseases they developed.

The findings were disturbing. Those students whose psychological tests showed they could not externalize their feelings—those who kept things bottled up inside—developed fatal cancer of all types later in life at an increased incidence.[6] In sum, Dr. Thomas's findings seemed to indicate that being a medical student could be life-threatening, since medical schools in general foster the internalization of feelings that correlated with the development of cancer.

Her study forced me to recall my own experiences in medical school and the years of internship and residency training that followed. The conditions I knew, despite a few improvements, remain largely the same today. In most if not all medical schools and post-graduate training programs, students soon discover that "keeping things inside" is a way to get ahead. Expressing emotion—candidly saying what one feels, getting it out, being one's own person—is frowned upon. Instead, machismo is valued—a silent, masculine, "I can take it" attitude in which one never complains no matter how difficult the work load. Following medical school the pressure to suffer quietly and withhold emotional expression intensifies. Intern and residency programs are widely viewed as a rite of passage that one must endure without complaining in spite of hard work, inhumane hours, low pay, chronic fatigue, and sleep deprivation.

In addition, there is the "dirty little secret" of medical student abuse and harassment, which many schools pretend does not exist. This abuse goes beyond overwork, sleep deprivation, and low pay to verbal, physical, psychological, sexual, and racial abuse, as well as to doctors being placed at unnecessary medical risk and to various forms of intimidation.[7] The way most students cope with this treatment is simply to endure it quietly. Thus from the earliest stages of medical school to the completion of postgraduate training, the psychological strategy of keeping things inside and holding one's tongue is encouraged.

Clearly, students' statements such as those that opened this chapter cannot be dismissed as comments from a few disgruntled "complainers." There is plenty of statistical evidence to the contrary. At one major medical school, 80 percent of seniors reported being abused during their training, and more than two-thirds stated that at least one of the episodes was of "major importance and very upsetting." Sixteen percent of the students surveyed said the abuse would "always affect them."[8]

Today the Thomas study does not stand alone. It has stimulated many researchers to try to unravel the particular mechanisms involved in the increased cancer incidence in medical students. One example comes from Ohio State University Medical Center, where researcher Ronald Glaser and his co-workers took blood samples from medical students at various times during the school year. They found that the students' immune systems worked less well at exam time. The activity of natural killer cells, which kill cancer cells, was impaired, and other types of cells produced less interferon, a chemical important in the immune response. Glaser also asked the medical students to keep tabs on minor symptoms such as coughs and colds that limited their activity. As predicted, these were greater during exam time, when their immune systems worked less well.

For many, being a "good student" may be similar to the experience of being a "good patient" described in the preceding chapter. They may be victims of a perpetual sense of "no exit" or impasse. They may realize at some level their need for greater emotional expression but be burdened by overwhelming pressures to conform. This may seem utterly odd to an outside observer, who may think that medical students are on top of the world, in total control of their destiny with nothing but security and success ahead. But medical students can be some of the most driven members of our society. For many of them, becoming a doctor is not a self-chosen path but a veritable form of enslavement to the expectations of family and their own unconscious desires for success, power, and approval. Students who are subject to these psychological stresses begin to resemble the "patient patient" whose life is threatened but who has no acceptable course of action. The student may want to escape, but the pressures will not allow it. In this situation, the student's emotions turn inward as he or she tacitly agrees to "grin and bear it." As Thomas's research suggests, the target organ of this inward emotional trajectory can be the immune system, with the eventual development of fatal cancer.

Although these risks are real, statistical findings should not be considered a sentence for having an immune system that someday will fail. After all, most of the medical students in Thomas' study did *not* develop fatal cancers. And these findings certainly do not apply to the student who discovers healthy ways to participate in medical school, as many do.

Our purpose in examining the health threats faced by medical students is not to pillory medical schools, but to look at the effect on health of the perceived *meaning* of one's situation. Anyone can see that the problems of medical students are not unique to them. They could be matched by students at other kinds of schools or by employees on various sorts of jobs. In fact, "medical student" may be considered a metaphor applying to anyone who feels unhappily trapped in an occupation in which expression is intensely restricted, whether or not abuse or harassment is involved. The consequences of being stuck in such a position seem similar, regardless of the specific occupation: poorer health and an increased fatality rate.

Why? We observed earlier that *job satisfaction* has been shown to be the best predictor of first heart attacks—better than the classical risk factors of smoking, blood pressure, or cholesterol, which *are not present* in most persons under fifty at the time of their first heart attack. We saw that persons having no control over their work loads—waiters, gas station attendants, certain data processors—have an increased incidence of sudden death. We observed that more heart attacks occur on Monday than any other day of the week, and that they cluster around nine in the morning, the beginning of the workweek. All these findings suggest that the emotions that surround our work role are crucial to our health. When they take the form of chronic despair, no control, and a sense of impasse, the stage is set for major health problems.

If medical students have a different emotional pattern—if they demonstrate excessive hostility instead of suppression of emotion—their pattern of disease differs. In a study done over a twenty-five-year period at the University of North Carolina Medical School, a battery of psychological tests were given to all entering medical students. Researchers found that students measuring high in "hostility" faced four times the risk of heart disease later in life, and a six-fold increase in mortality risk.[9]

Although we will look at specific examples of how people can escape difficult life situations in Part III, "Healing Breakthroughs," we can note here that no job or stressful situation has absolute power over anyone. Psychologist Suzanne Kobasa has investigated why some people wither under a stressful occupation while others thrive. She studied lawyers because of their popular image of thriving on stress, working at a strenuous pace, seldom getting sick, and living long lives. In one study of 157 lawyers in general practice, her research team found that many had undergone frequent changes at work, including hiring and firing of staff and salary adjustments, and severe off-the-job stresses such as deaths in families, separations, and divorces. However, no correlation could be found between any of these events and their physical health. The researchers discovered that a powerful role was played by the attorneys' attitude and beliefs. Those who were convinced of the importance, purpose, and intrinsic value of their work had the fewest symptoms such as headaches, nervousness, and insomnia. Kobasa proposed that many attorneys may have developed the ability to thrive on stress because they *believed* they were expected to do so.[10]

Psychologist Blair Justice affirms Kobasa's suggestion that, to a great degree, "thinking makes it so." In his excellent book *Who Gets Sick: Thinking and Health,* he states, "Our attitudes . . . toward the very subject of stress can influence our reactions when we are in trying situations. Our physiological responses will be considerably less intense if we see stress as an inevitable part of life and a challenge rather than something that is awful and must be avoided."[11]

Psychologist Viktor Frankl, who survived the Nazi death camps in World War II, understood the protective, lifesaving effects of a sense of purpose. In his book *Man's Search for Meaning,* he stated, "Those who know how close the connection is between the state of a man—his courage and hope, or lack of them—and the state of . . . his body will understand that the sudden loss of hope and courage can have a deadly effect."[12]

Despair comes in many forms. While we might avoid many of these experiences, some of them are ubiquitous. Next we look at one of the most powerful and most common forms of despair: the loss of a mate.

Broken Hearts:
The Toxicity of Bereavement

The love we have in our youth is superficial compared to the love that an old man has for his old wife.

—WILL DURANT

The concept that a person can die from being separated suddenly
from a loved one is rooted in history and spans all cultures. One of
the most vivid descriptions of this phenomenon comes from David
Livingstone, the Scottish physician and missionary. Livingstone
explored central Africa when the slave trade was flourishing, and he
left this account, as recorded in his excellent biography by Tim Jeal:

". . . the strangest disease I have seen in this country seems
really to be brokenheartedness, and it attacks free men who
have been captured and made slaves."
    Many recently captured men seemed to waste away and
die within weeks for no obvious physical cause. Livingstone
talked to many of those in the first stages of this inexplicable
disease, and wrote: "They ascribed their only pain to the
heart, and placed the hand correctly on the spot."[1]

The ties that develop in many marital relationships simply defy
description and sometimes seem surreal. Customary words such as
"love," "intimacy," and "bondedness" are inadequate to describe

them. These connections are so profound that the physical welfare of one partner can affect that of the other, even across great distances.

Consider what happened one summer morning to Arthur Severn, a distinguished landscape painter, and his wife, Joan. The following account was collected by John Ruskin (1819–1900), the English writer, art critic, and social reformer:

> Leaving his wife asleep in bed one morning, Mr. Arthur Severn decided to go down to the lake for an early sail. Then, at about 7 A.M., Mrs. Severn awoke with a start.
>
> "I [felt] I had had a hard blow on my mouth," she said, "and with a distinct sense that I had been cut and was bleeding under my upper lip." She grabbed a handkerchief to absorb the blood, and was surprised to find none. Finally she was able to return to sleep.
>
> When her husband returned for breakfast at 9:30, she noticed he was purposefully sitting farther away from her than usual and seemed to be hiding something. Every now and then he would put his handkerchief furtively to his lip, just as she had done earlier.
>
> "Arthur, why are you doing that? . . . I know you have hurt yourself!" she said.
>
> He responded, ". . . when I was sailing, a sudden squall came, throwing the tiller suddenly round, and it struck me a bad blow in the mouth, under the upper lip, and it has been bleeding a good deal and won't stop."
>
> Mrs. Severn then announced her experience which happened at about the same time, ". . . much to his surprise, and all who were with us at breakfast."[2]

Spouses frequently seem to "just know" that something is wrong or is about to happen to their partner, as in the following two case histories:

> My husband is manager of a large ice cream factory located almost three miles away. He usually came home from work between 11:00 P.M. and 6:00 A.M., and I was never worried when he was late.
>
> One night, expecting him to be late, I settled down to watch television but could not. Feeling something must be wrong, I unsuccessfully tried phoning my husband three times. At 2:00 A.M. I decided to

walk to the factory. The door was locked and there was no reply. Feeling even more uneasy, for no apparent reason, I decided to break a window and climb in. I found my husband locked in the cold storage (walk-in) refrigerator, and on comparing notes discovered he'd been locked in it only minutes before I felt the need to call him for the first time.[3]

In 1949 my husband left our home in Dallas, Texas, on a business trip, which involved traveling from Boston to Washington by plane. After he left I had a feeling I would not see him alive again. I felt he should not take the plane from Boston to Washington, and I could hardly wait until the next day to call him. When I finally reached him I begged him not to do so. It turned out that he did not have to go to Washington after all. Although he had reservations for the flight, he canceled at the last minute. The change in plans saved his life, for, approaching the Washington airport, the plane was struck by another aircraft and crashed into the Potomac River, killing all on board.[4]

These stories indicate the profound connectedness that can occur between husband and wife. I believe these deep connections are extraordinarily commonplace and have discovered that many couples can match these cases with similar stories of their own. It is important to acknowledge this intimacy, because unless we do we cannot properly understand one of our most traumatic and frequently fatal experiences: the despair and bereavement following the death of a spouse.

In almost every study done in the Western world to look at these effects, the mortality of the surviving spouse during the first year of bereavement has been found to be two to twelve times that of married persons the same age. In the United States 700,000 persons aged fifty or more lose their spouses annually. Of these, 35,000 die during the first year of grief. Researcher Steven Schleifer of New York's Mount Sinai Hospital calculates that 20 percent, or 7,000, of these deaths are directly caused by the loss of the spouse.[5]

Why should the death of a spouse be so devastating? The above cases suggest that many couples function at a certain psychological level as a single entity. Thoughts and feelings are more than "shared" in the ordinary sense; there seems to be a literal *union* of the two psyches that operates in spite of physical separation. It is possible that this felt sense of union sets the stage for catastrophic mind-body effects when either husband or wife dies. Once so immediate and sustaining, the bond is now broken, and for the survivor life may not seem worth living. Or the survivor may even experience a desire to reestablish the connection by joining the deceased in death; as Sir Henry Wootton put it,

> He first deceased; she for a little tried
> To live without him; liked it not, and died.

In 1967 psychiatrists Thomas Holmes and Richard Rahe of the University of Washington developed a simple scale for measuring the impact on health of various life events. They extracted a list of happenings in the life charts of about 5,000 medical patients, boiled them down to forty-three common events, and assigned weights to both positive and negative experiences. They found that the most traumatic event of all—the one most likely to have injurious effects on one's health—was the death of a spouse.[6]

A typical study showing these effects was done in 1967, in the small rural Welsh community of Llanidloes (population 2,350), by researchers W. D. Rees and S. G. Lutkins. Between 1960 and 1965, 371 residents of Llanidloes had died. Rees and Lutkins contacted 903 close relatives of these deceased persons, "close relative" meaning a spouse, a child, a parent, or a sibling. They found that 5 percent of the surviving close relatives died within the first year of the death of their loved one, compared to 0.7 percent of persons of the same age in the community who had not lost a loved one. This meant there was a *sevenfold* increase in the death rate for surviving close relatives during the first year of bereavement.

The place where the person died was also important. If the death took place in a hospital, the death rate in the survivors was "only" doubled; but if the death occurred some place other than the home or the hospital (e.g., on a road or in a field), the risk of death of surviving close relatives was *five* times higher.[7]

One of the most incisive looks at the medical importance of closeness between human beings is psychologist James J. Lynch's book *The Broken Heart: The Medical Consequences of Loneliness.* Lynch's work leaves no doubt that when our ties with each other are broken, the consequences can be as real as a heart attack, cancer, or stroke. Yet we have hidden our eyes to the biological consequences of severing these ties. As Lynch states,

> The real cost of a deep personal love for another human being can only be seen in the shattering loss that is felt when that love is suddenly and permanently taken away. This idea is not new. A few hundred years ago "grief" was openly recognized as a cause of death. Today, however, a broken heart would never be listed as a cause of death in any U.S. hospital. We have grown far too "medically wise" to tolerate such an ill-defined diagnosis. Patients now die of atherosclerosis, ventricular fibrillation, or congestive heart failure brought on by age, damaged hearts and arteries, or poor eating habits.[8]

Closeness between humans is not just a learned behavior; it has biological roots as well. Studies in primates show that if the normal mothering process is interrupted by isolating the mother and infant from each other, the infant's brain does not develop normally. For example, the number and the sensitivity of the infant brain's receptor sites for endorphins—the internal morphinelike chemicals that affect mood—are diminished.[9]

In all mammalian species, if the mother and infant are separated the infant emits some type of distress cry, which evokes complementary behaviors in the mother. Again, studies in a variety of species suggest a relationship between endorphins and this mother-infant bond. If one blocks the receptor sites for endorphins by giving a certain chemical, the need for social attachment is increased; and if one gives morphine in very low doses, this need is diminished, as both the distress call of the infant and the response of the mother are abolished.[10]

An example of the biological consequences of broken bonds and isolation early in life is the legendary story of Frederick II, ruler of Sicily in the thirteenth century, retold by Lynch in *The Broken Heart*. Frederick believed that all men were born with a common language, presumably an ancient one such as Hebrew. To test his theory, he separated newborn infants from their natural mothers and gave them to foster mothers. He commanded these foster mothers to care for babies physically but never to speak to them, in order to learn what language they would naturally speak. The experiment was a failure— all the children died.[11]

The innate need for closeness is especially obvious in the behavior of small children, who will go to almost unbelievable lengths to maintain it. Even when parents become sources of danger, as in instances of child abuse or neglect, children will continue to maneuver psychologically to maintain the sense of a safe attachment. Even when abused they will blame themselves instead of their parents, in order to perpetuate the illusion of security and closeness. Studies in other species show that the young, just like human children, will actually *increase* their attachment to the parent when faced with a threat originating from the parent, and even when the parent has ceased to provide nurture and protection.

How does the despair we feel during bereavement actually affect the body? Part of the answer comes from the work of Steven J. Schleifer and his colleagues at New York's Mount Sinai Hospital. Schleifer studied the immune function of fifteen men whose wives had terminal breast cancer. Of interest were the T- and B-lymphocytes, the body's two main immune cells. Prior to the death of the wife, the researchers found that these cells functioned normally. But beginning shortly after the wife's death, and extending for many months in the period of grief, the cells, though normal in number, stopped working. They could not even be made to work when extracted from the blood of the men and exposed in test tubes to chemicals that ordinarily "turn them on."[12]

It is often argued that emotions such as "despair," "grief," and "bereavement" cannot account for these findings, because physical effects demand physical, not mental, causes. Perhaps despairing, bereaved persons simply take poorer care of themselves. Maybe they tend to neglect their diet and medical care and to take medications incorrectly, just as they are more likely to commit suicide. But these are only partial explanations. In the end, it is the felt emotion that is fundamental. After all, the gun used in the suicide does not pull its own trigger. Neither does the grieving person's food refuse to be eaten. One may install any number of intervening variables between the loss of the spouse and the death of the grieving survivor, but in the end one runs out of physical behaviors and into the emotions and the meaning of the broken bond.

Schleifer's study showing failed immunity during bereavement does not stand alone. Researchers in Sydney, Australia, in 1977 studied the immune activity in twenty-six persons two and six weeks after their spouses died. At both times the bereaved showed reduced immune activity when compared to a control group.[13]

There is evidence that loneliness itself can reduce immune function, even when bereavement is not involved. When seventy-six first-year medical students at Ohio State University were studied, those who had the highest loneliness scores and highest stress on psychological tests had the lowest levels of NK (natural killer) cells. Students having the highest level of NK cells, in contrast, had the lowest loneliness scores.[14]

The *meaning* to the individual of being alone appears to be a crucial factor in determining the effects of social isolation. In 1986 Peggy Reynolds and George A. Kaplan, epidemiologists with the California Department of Health Services, reported their findings on the relationship between cancer and social isolation. Employing data from an earlier study of nearly 7,000 healthy adults in Alameda County, California, they discovered that socially isolated women had a significantly greater chance of developing and dying from cancer. But it wasn't only social isolation in terms of lack of social contacts that was important, they reported, but the *perception* or the *feeling* of loneliness—in other words, what being alone *meant* to them. Women who had many social contacts but *felt* isolated had 2.4 times the normal risk of dying from hormone-related cancers (breast, uterine, and ovarian). And those women who had few social contacts *and* felt isolated were *five* times as likely to die from such cancers. Interestingly, social ties did not seem to affect whether men got cancer in general, but among those who developed cancer, death was sooner in those who were socially isolated.[15]

Sometimes the effects of separation are sudden in onset. A dramatic and poignant example cited by Lynch is the near-simultaneous death of female twins:[16]

As young adults living in North Carolina, the twins were extremely close to each other. Neither had married and they had never been separated for any significant period of time. In their early twenties they began to experience psychological changes such as flattening of affect and emotions, loss of social interest, disturbed sleep and appetite, and the development of suspicions and delusions. This led to a diagnosis of schizophrenia, and in spite of valiant attempts by their parents to care for them at home for more than a decade, it became necessary to hospitalize them from time to time in a mental facility. Eventually the parents gave up their struggle to maintain them outside the hospital and the twins were admitted for the final time on April 1, 1962.

Following admission to the institution they refused to eat and became increasingly isolated socially. They would not interact with the staff and would answer questions with only the most minimal responses. The staff came to believe they were reinforcing each other's behavior with negative attitudes, and in an attempt to treat them more successfully the decision was made to separate them and house them in distant parts of the facility.

A tragic series of events immediately took place. Following the first evening of their separation they went to bed as usual. At 10:20 P.M., 11:30 P.M., and 12:00 midnight the staff routinely checked them, finding them both sleeping with normal respiratory movements. However, on the next check at 12:45 A.M., twin A was found dead. This prompted an immediate investigation of twin B, who was also found dead.

The patient who shared the room with twin B told an interesting story about the circumstances immediately preceding her death. Twin B had stood looking longingly out of the window of her dormitory, gazing up at the room window where her sister was housed. This was not considered unusual behavior by her roommate, who was accustomed to seeing patients behave like this. Shortly thereafter she was found dead.

But how could twin B have known that twin A had died? Could there have been—as in the stories at the beginning of this chapter—some extraordinary form of communication between them despite their physical separation?

In a previous book, *Recovering the Soul,* I explored evidence that all minds are interconnected and cannot ultimately be separated—that they are neither confined to points in space such as brains and bodies, nor to points in time such as the present moment or even single lifetimes; that they are, in a word, *nonlocal.*[17] Thus, while "separation" applies to physical bodies, it may not apply to minds. This would mean that minds are ultimately not bounded, having no fundamental barriers between them; and if unbounded, they are unitary and in some sense one. This possibility has been affirmed by Erwin Schrödinger, one of the greatest physicists of our time, who boldly stated, "Mind is by its very nature a *singulare tantum*. I should say: the over-all number of minds is just one."[18] If this is the case, the twins were not really separated mentally, only physically, and twin B indeed might have known that her sister had died because they were "of one mind."

If minds are in some sense single and unitary, this would mean that the sense of total separation and aloneness that comes with bereavement is in a part a delusion. But if it is a delusion, why is bereavement frequently fatal? For one thing, as we've seen, the need for closeness is not just "in the mind," it is rooted in our biology, and the body responds to aloneness with automatic, reflexlike actions. Moreover, our thoughts do not have to be true to affect the body; illusion can be as potent as truth.

We can recall that in voodoo, which is one of the most dramatic examples of the fatal effects of a false belief, the hexed person wills himself to death out of the belief that he had been completely separated from his society. This situation may apply to many bereaved persons. If their will to join the deceased is strong enough, this may serve to cut them off from the land of the living. As in the voodoo situation, the body may comply and die.

If we deeply sensed that separation cannot in principle be final, bereavement would not cease to exist but its effects might well be attenuated. This could mean that many of the 7,000 annual deaths that are estimated to be a direct consequence of bereavement might be avoided.

In this and the preceding chapters we have dwelled only on how the breakdown of meaning affects our health. If these tragic tales were the whole story, this would be a meager harvest. But they are only the beginning. Now we leave the shadow side of meanings and emotions to see eventually that they can be life creating, spiritually sustaining, and a vital force in healing.

But before we look at the ways meaning works its magic in health, we first must take a crucial step: we must allow the physical body to take on new meaning by daring to see it in a new way.

PART TWO

NEW MEANING, NEW BODY

Science . . . at first sight seems to have no special platform for man, mind, or meaning. Man? Pure biochemistry! Mind? Memory modelable by electronic circuitry! Meaning? Why ask after that puzzling and intangible commodity?

. . . What is man that the universe should be mindful of him? . . . is not man an unimportant bit of dust on an unimportant planet in an unimportant galaxy in an unimportant region somewhere in the vastness of space?

No! The philosopher of old was right! Meaning is important, even central.

—JOHN ARCHIBALD WHEELER[1]

Meaning Links Mind and Matter:
The Theory of Physicist David Bohm

> I wish to bring out a new way of thinking, consistent
> with modern physics, that does not divide mind
> from matter or subject from object. . . . Meaning,
> which is simultaneously mental and physical, can
> serve as the link or bridge between realms. . . .
> This link is indivisible.
>
> —DAVID BOHM[1]

Imagine: You are walking down a dark alley, all alone after the late-night movie, taking a shortcut to get to the subway station. Suddenly a figure appears in the distant shadows, walking slowly toward you. The closer it gets, the more sinister and menacing it appears. You are fearful, your heart begins to pound, and panic floods your entire being. You start to run when suddenly the shadowy figure raises an arm and shouts, "Hi! Need a ride?" Sick with fear, you recognize your friend from work who must have been at the same movie. The terror slowly subsides and you feel your body's emergency responses coming back to normal. You are face to face with your friend now, in control of your emotions, as you turn and walk with him toward his car.

The "shadow in the alley" story is used by physicist David Bohm in his theory of *soma-significance* to illustrate the role of meaning in how reality unfolds for us. *Soma* comes from a Greek word meaning "the body" and is customarily used to refer to the physical body as opposed to the spirit. *Significance,* on the other hand, is connected with the mind. It is derived from the Latin *significans,* "that which is signified; meaning."[2] By juxtaposing these two words Bohm suggests a connection between the body and the mind, the material and the mental. And the connection between the two, he proposes, is through a third entity, *meaning.*[3]

Yet the connecting link of meaning is not a physical thing like a bridge connecting two land masses that is different from the elements it connects. Rather, all three entities—mind, body, and meaning—are inseparable and form a whole.

As a common example of how apparently separate entites can really be a whole in disguise, Bohm cites the magnet. We ordinarily think of a magnet as having two separate parts, a north and a south pole. But the poles aren't really separate, because one could not exist without the other. And they are encompassed or bridged by a magnetic field which, although it also has a separate name and sounds different from the poles, shares an overall wholeness with them. The bridge (the magnetic field) and the elements it connects (the two poles) cannot be understood separately. So it is the whole, not the parts, that is fundamental.

Now back to the dark alley and the shadowy, threatening figure who eventually proved to be a friend. Our soma (our body's responses) were obviously tied to our psyche (our emotions), and the bridge between them was the *significance* or the *meaning* we drew. As the meanings changed, our soma and the psychological experience changed as well. Like the magnet's north and south poles and its magnetic field, our three elements—mind, body, and meaning—were also an inseparable whole.

But *how* did our meanings in the dark alley make our heart pound and our palms sweaty? These connections occur, says Bohm, through well-known biochemical processes occurring in the body and brain:

each particular kind of significance is carried by some somatic order, arrangement, connection, and organization of distinguishable elements. . . . Modern scientific studies strongly indicate that . . . meanings are carried somatically by . . . physical, chemical, and electrical processes into the brain and the rest of the nervous system, where they are apprehended at higher and higher intellectual and emotional levels of meaning.[4]

This is a way of saying that meanings are not simply reflected in the workings of the body, they in some sense *are* the body just as they in some sense *are* the mind.

Bohm suggests that mind, matter, and meaning have a genuine ontological similarity and are not immiscible entities that are working *on* each other. This places the problem of the interaction of mind and body on a different footing. Because, contrary to the view in the West, they intrinsically are not different, their interaction makes sense and the problem of visualizing how mind and body might interact abates.

It is only a short jump from the dark alley to the many case histories in this book. Whether we are talking about the fear of unknown shadows or the fear of surgery, the same processes are involved. *Any* meaning-rich emotion—whether hopelessness, panic, depression, anxiety, or suffering, or courage, joy, exultation, or ecstasy—is connected to our bodies through a similar overall process in which meaning plays a key role.

Sometimes it seems that meaning has no role whatsoever to play in health and illness, and that Bohm's theory of soma-significance breaks down. In trauma or in cases of children born with genetic diseases, where does meaning enter? These problems seem overwhelmingly physical, with meanings and the mind nowhere in sight. Bohm acknowledges that reality may indeed present itself to us in ways that seem genuinely physical. But he maintains that even in these instances the wholeness of matter, mind, and meaning is unbroken. As he puts it,

there is only one "field" of reality as a whole, containing the universal but relative distinction between generalized soma [matter] and generalized significance [mind] . . . which . . . are not separate substances. . . . What we call "matter" is then encountered wherever the somatic side of this universal and fundamental distinction is the major factor and what we call "mind" is encountered wherever the side of the significance is the major factor. . . . Perhaps both sides ultimately meet at "infinite" depths, on a ground from which the whole of existence emerges.[5]

The world, according to Bohm, is a chimera and has different ways of showing itself. Sometimes we see the physical, sometimes the mental side more prominently. In both cases the whole is still there, and meaning remains the connecting principle uniting the two. Even in an overtly physical illness such as a broken leg, we still experience meanings which, through the unending feedback processes of the body, influence healing by affecting factors such as blood flow and inflammation. Even in genetically based diseases, meaning is still part of the experience and feeds back to some extent on the "physical" problem as will be seen in the case of congenital ichthyosis successfully treated with hypnosis (page 151).

Bohm's theory of soma-significance is complemented by his *signa-somatic* theory, which is simply the matter-mind interrelationship working from the direction of the mind. Just as the body's reactions can affect our perceptions (the soma is significant: "soma-significance"), mental factors can generate changes in our body (meanings are significant: "signa-somatic"). These two theories are "the loop" flowing in different directions, the flip side of each other.

Other eminent thinkers have taken positions similar to Bohm's. For example, Alfred North Whitehead stated:

neither physical nature nor life can be understood unless we fuse them together as essential factors in the composition of the "really real" whose interconnections and individual characters constitute the universe. . . . Scientific reasoning is completely dominated by the presupposition that mental functionings are not properly part of nature. . . . This sharp distinction between mentality and nature has no ground in our fundamental observation. . . . All [the] functionings of nature influence each other, require each other, and lead on to each other. . . . The human individual is one fact, body and mind. . . . We are in the world and the world is in us.[6]

Whitehead's view is hardly distinguishable from the following comment of Bohm:

One can see that ultimately the soma-significant (the physical) and the signa-somatic (the mental) process extends even into the environment. . . . Even relationships with Nature and with the Cosmos are evidently deeply affected by what these mean to us. In turn, such meanings fundamentally affect our actions toward them, and thus indirectly their actions back on us are influenced in a similar way. Indeed, insofar as we know it, are aware of it, and can act on it, the whole of Nature, including our civilization which has evolved from Nature and is still a part of Nature, is one movement that is both soma-significant and signa-somatic.[7]

These perspectives are similar to those of another seminal thinker of our century, anthropologist and philosopher Gregory Bateson:

Mind is not "something" separate from nature. It is identical at various levels of order with all of nature, not solely with individual brains. It emerges as a characteristic of processes of nature at a certain level of evolution. It is therefore futile to look for evidence of mental process as located purely in the brain of an individual organism. We must look for such evidence in the entire network of patterns of interaction which that organism has with its environment, or which a group or society of organisms has with its environment. . . . The individual mind is immanent but not only in the body. It is immanent also in the pathways and messages outside the body.[8]

A few physicists such as Bohm believe that meaning must be recognized as a legitimate concept in physics. If it proves necessary to include meaning as a factor in order to understand simple systems such as atoms, it seems likely that meaning also will be crucial in understanding the behavior of much more complex entities such as human beings. And if this approach is applied to medicine, a great historical loop will have closed and meaning—once regarded as a vital factor in getting well—will again have a home in healing.

Now our journey into meaning takes us to an area that is usually our first concern in health: the human body.

The Body as Machine

Let us conclude boldly then, that man is a machine.

—JULIEN OFFRAY DE LA METTRIE, 1750
Man: A Machine[1]

In 1847 the Materialist Manifesto—a statement that all life processes would eventually be explained in terms of physical and chemical events—was issued by a group of European scientists. It contains the following statement from the famous materialist scientist, duBois-Reymond:

> "Brücke and I have sworn to make prevail the truth that in the organism no other forces are effective than the purely physical-chemical. . . ."[2]

What is a body? The answers humans have given to this question have varied tremendously throughout history. Philosopher–social critic Ivan Illich states that, prior to the fifteenth and sixteenth centuries, Europeans did not regard bodies as objects separate from the person or personality. This was particularly obvious in their attitude toward corpses, which were treated almost like living individuals by the law. The dead could sue and be sued by the living, and criminal proceedings against the dead were common. Illich gives examples of such attitudes and their ongoing influence:

Pope Urban VIII, who had been poisoned by his successor, was dug up, solemnly judged a simonist, had his right hand cut off, and was thrown into the Tiber. After being hanged as a thief, a man might still have his head cut off for being a traitor. The dead could also be called to witness. The widow could still repudiate her husband by putting the keys and his purse on his casket. Even today the executor acts in the name of the dead, and we still speak of the "desecration" of a grave or the secularization of a public cemetery when it is turned into a park.[3]

Our attitudes toward the body continue to evolve. Some of the interesting current ideas come from science fiction writers. Novelist Naomi Mitchison has proposed connections between mental processes and the shape of the body. She describes a fabulous race of beings who are highly intelligent and whose bodies have six arms and radial symmetry, like starfish. Because their bodies have no right or left, these beings do not think in terms of polar opposites like "right" or "wrong," "black" or "white," but shades of gray. For them, these absolute categories are absurd simplifications and simply make no sense. They are thus well equipped to handle complex thoughts such as paradox.[4]

Is there a connection between the shape of our bodies and how we think? Alastair J. Cunningham, a researcher with the Ontario Cancer Institute in Toronto, believes the answer may be yes. He proposes that we humans, perhaps because of our bilateral symmetry, have an "all or nothing" approach to causality, and experience difficulty understanding the many complex interacting systems that have become important to us in economics, politics, and ecology. Medicine is particularly affected by our preference for "all or nothing" approaches. We search incessantly for "the" cure for diseases, hoping to find the "magic bullet" that will cure cancer or a single factor that causes AIDS.[5]

Whether or not corpses should be treated as persons, and whether or not the actual shape of our body affects how we think, one thing is certain: our images, thoughts, emotions, and attitudes *about* our bodies exert profound effects on our health and healing.

BODY ILLUSIONS

If our image of our body is so important, we ought to make sure we "get it right." But even today, when we pride ourselves on being scientific, on having discarded antiquated views such as the living corpse, our body images are almost never accurate. In fact, they reflect colossal errors. Consider the following examples:

- *The Solid Body*. This is one of our most unquestioned assumptions. If I pinch or poke my body, it resists, it pushes back. But in fact, the solid body is an illusion. While the body does have a certain mass—we can weigh it and document a certain "heaviness"—it is almost totally thin air. Almost all the mass in the atoms of the body is concentrated in the nuclei. All the rest of the atom is emptiness, except for a few electrons which are separated from the nucleus by vast reaches of empty space. To get an idea of this immensity, imagine an orange in the center of the Astrodome. This gives a relative picture of the "stuff" of the body; almost all of it is "nothing."

  Our ordinary assumptions about matter are archaic. Modern physics reveals that matter is not the hard, enduring stuff we commonly think, not the indivisible atoms postulated by the ancient Greeks such as Democritus. Atoms are today conceived as waves of probability, not billiard balls, BBs, or pellets. Perhaps, some physicists say, the dynamic properties of matter depend on us and the observations we make. Maybe we have a hand in shaping the world and the stuff of our bodies—a world we once presumed was completely independent of ourselves.

- *The Stable Body*. Again, an illusion. Your body at this instant is not the body you had when you started reading this book, and it will not be the body you have when you finish it. The body's atoms are always being replaced in an invisible stream. Each year, 98 percent of the 10^{28} atoms in the body are replaced; at the end of five years *all* are renewed, down to the very last one.[6]

- *The Individual Body.* A wrong assumption again. Bodies are incessantly mixing with other bodies through the endless shuttle of atoms just mentioned. Writer Guy Murchie has calculated that, given a few assumptions such as uniform mixing of the air, each breath we take has millions of molecules breathed recently by each and every one of the five billion people on the earth.[7] And the molecules have been breathed not just by people, but by *any* living thing that breathes—cows, horses, snakes, spiders, birds, bees, and so forth. These molecules actually become the stuff of the body. This means that remnants of the bodies of Lao-tzu, Jesus, Mohammed, Buddha—and also Hitler, Genghis Khan, and Stalin—are entering you and everyone else.

- *The Terrestrial Body.* We ordinarily think we had our origins in the ovum of our mother and the sperm of our father. But with the exception of primordial hydrogen, which has been around since the Big Bang occurred some fourteen billion years ago, all the stuff in our bodies originated not in the DNA of our parents but in the interior of stars, a minimum of a billion years ago. These stars eventually exploded after cooking their ingredients, spewing them into space. The planets were formed out of this material, and our bodies eventually came into being. Thus we have our origins in the stars—this is not mystical or poetic observation but scientific fact.

- *The Stationary Body.* As I sit here, writing this book, my body seems still. But if I had some gadget capable of mapping the path my body is inscribing in space at each moment, the pattern would be "giddy and highly complicated," as Lincoln Barnett, one of Einstein's biographers, put it. Barnett describes our motions:

> In addition to its daily rotation about its axis at the rate of 1000 miles an hour, and its annual revolution about the sun at the rate of 20 miles a second, the earth is also involved in a number of other less familiar gyrations. Contrary to popular belief the

moon does not revolve around the earth; they revolve around each other—or more precisely, around
a common center of gravity. The entire solar system,
moreover, is moving within the local star system at
the rate of 13 miles a second; the local star system
is moving within the Milky Way at the rate of 200
miles a second; and the whole Milky Way is drifting
with respect to the remote external galaxies at the rate
of 100 miles a second—and all in different directions![8]

All these three-dimensional arabesques are taking place
in a universe so large that, since the Big Bang, our galaxy
has made only twenty trips around the circuit.

• *The Mindless Body.* For over three hundred years Western
civilization has regarded all matter, including the body, as
mindless. With the advent of modern science, however, the
mind has come to be regarded as a special, sole property of
the brain. Recently, this idea, too, has come under fire, as
body tissues and organs distant from the brain have been
discovered to possess brainlike properties. For instance, the
endorphins, those celebrated chemicals that affect our mental life by influencing our moods, were originally thought
present only in the brain. Now, however, they are known
to be produced in many body parts including various types
of white blood cells and the gastrointestinal tract. Not only
do these sites make endorphins, they have receptors for
them as well. Thus a network seems to be in place for
actual communication between the brain and these distant
sites. What is implied by the brainlike properties of these
body parts? Do they, like the brain "have mind"? This
possibility has seriously been raised by Candace B. Pert,
former chief of brain chemistry at the National Institute of
Mental Health. Pert has said "I can no longer make a strong
distinction between the brain and the body,"[9] and sees in
research findings a "need to start thinking about how
consciousness can be projected into various parts of the
body."[10] In the wake of these developments, the old idea
that the body is mindless seems increasingly illusory.

Our illusions regarding the body—that it is mindless and purposeless, that it behaves essentially like a machine—have paved the way for the loss of meaning in health and illness. Yet for almost the entire history of civilization, meaning has been an essential part of healing. Even today, when *most* people on the face of the earth become ill, they are treated not in modern hospitals nor by physicians but by the folk healer, the shaman, the medicine man. For them, meaning is utterly essential in understanding their illness. Without knowing what a disease means, rational therapy cannot be chosen and "cure" is unthinkable. Against this backdrop, the modern attitude that disease means nothing is a genuine aberration on the world scene, a strange interlude in the history of healing.

What happened? How did meaning become a pariah in modern medicine? Often I have tried to put myself in the place of the physicians who, a century or two ago, were involved in turning medicine away from meaning and have tried to imagine what that transition must have been like. I do not believe these clinician-scientists were cold and uncaring, as physicians are frequently depicted today, or that they failed to find meaning in their own lives. The loss of meaning must surely have been a subtle process—a gradual weaning, a slow fall. Meaning became less important, silently and invisibly, and was finally pushed aside altogether as physicians came to focus on other elements in the healing process—for instance, on the captivating idea that the entire universe, including the body, could be viewed as a machine.

THE BODY AS MACHINE

The physiologist Ludwig in the 1880s wrote a classic textbook PHYSIOLOGY which explained everything on one basis—mechanism. Later he was asked why he did not prepare a new edition of it. He said, "Such a work must be written by a young man; an old man is too well aware of his ignorance."

—LAWRENCE LESHAN[11]

In the midnineteenth century, one of the most distinguished physicians was the Irishman Robert James Graves. Graves was a legend in Britain and on the Continent.[12] In 1835 he described in the *London Medical and Surgical Journal* an illness that bears his name to this day—Graves's disease, a syndrome characterized by protuberant eyes and an enlarged, overactive thyroid gland.

But thirteen years later, this contribution was dwarfed by a simple act Robert James Graves performed—an act that, although now almost forgotten, decisively influenced the way we view the human body. While standing at a patient's bedside, Graves advised *the timing of the pulse by a watch*.

The new technique quickly became standard. It seemed logical and affirmed further the notion that the whole of nature, including the human body, could be viewed as a complex machine. At the time that Graves took out his watch at the bedside of his patient, the Industrial Revolution had already made an indelible impression on medical thought. The midnineteenth-century physicians of England and Europe saw machines everywhere—the heart was a pump, the lungs were bellows, the limbs were pulleys and levers, the circulation was a sophisticated hydraulic system replete with valves, locks, and dams.

The machine metaphor fired their vision and, although we may now object to the metaphor, the vision was productive; today one stands in awe of the insights that rolled from the continental mind at an unbelievable rate. Advances in physical diagnosis, in particular, were notable. In the late eighteenth to the midnineteenth century, the art of the physical examination was being perfected, and many of the observations that make up today's textbooks date from that period. The powers of scrutiny of the physicians of that era seem ingenious in retrospect. We can only conclude from the detailed descriptions they left that we have lost something valuable today, when X rays, blood tests, and a myriad of other diagnostic tools have supplanted the eyes, ears, and hands of the physician. We doctors sometimes chide one another with, "If all else fails, do a physical exam; if that fails, take a history"—acknowledging that we have reversed in this technological, modern age the time-honored sequence of unraveling the mysteries of illness. The doctors of Graves's day, however, never put the cart before the horse. There were no fancy tests to tempt them, and their tools were crude at best. In spite of this—or perhaps because of it—the art of medicine evolved with great rapidity.

In the long shadow of the Industrial Revolution, many clinicians in addition to Graves made observations that burned into Western consciousness the notion that humans were entirely mechanical. Another example was the towering Sir Dominic John Corrigan, whose name is still familiar to every student of medicine. In 1832 he published an original description of aortic insufficiency, a condition wherein the aortic valve, which is situated at the junction of the heart's left ventricle and the aorta, becomes "insufficient" and allows blood to flow backward. As a result, the main pumping chamber of the heart, the left ventricle, has to pump an excessive volume of blood with each heartbeat, which it accomplishes with a forceful, exaggerated contraction. This is felt downstream as a sudden, heightened pulsation that immediately decreases or "falls off," since the pressure generated cannot be sustained because of the "leaky" aortic valve. Corrigan described this as a "water hammer" pulse, a term consistent with the machinelike view of the body. This term remains in use, along with the alternative name "Corrigan's pulse." Other machinelike metaphors gathered around the problem of the leaky aortic valve. For example, by listening carefully with a stethoscope over the femoral arteries in the groin, one can hear a booming noise called a "pistol-shot" sound.[13]

Even therapies took a machinelike flavor. Corrigan, for example, suggested that a flagging heart could be stimulated by tapping the chest with a hot spoon, and this procedure became known as "Corrigan's hammer."[14]

It is frequently argued that these picturesque metaphors are harmless enough. But they are not. They can convey meanings about the body that can be exceedingly potent and even destructive.

An example will show why. Hospital psychosis is a mental derangement in patients subjected to the rigors and trauma of being hospitalized for serious illness. A severe case of hospital psychosis occurred in a diabetic patient of mine whose body seemed to fall apart bit by bit. Originally admitted for a gangrenous toe, which was amputated, he experienced a heart attack after surgery. Then his entire foot on the other leg became gangrenous and had to be amputated. He then required an abdominal operation for a bowel obstruction. At this point the poor man developed horribly upsetting nightmares which invaded his waking life. He began to see his body as a failing, robotlike machine. It was clogged with rust and had parts falling off at random, for which nothing could be done. Recognizing the inevitable, the robot eventually began to participate in its own destruction by disassembling itself. In keeping with this vision, the man attempted to commit suicide. He survived the attempt and his experience. He deeply affected every nurse and physician who cared for him, for he became a mirror in which we recognized an uncomfortable truth: in many ways we *did* treat him and all patients as if they were machines, for we were trapped in our metaphors.

It is not only physicians who use metaphorical descriptions for the body and for illness. We *all* participate in metaphorical thinking when things go wrong with the body—and not only for cultural reasons but, more profoundly, because it is our nature to do so. Metaphors are an effort to understand the disease process, to make sense of what is happening.

As a medical student in the gynecology clinic, I witnessed a memorable example illustrating these points. A woman came with her husband to complain of "a mouse in [her] vagina." In addition to causing her severe pain, it would "bite" her husband during intercourse. They had endured this aggravation as long as possible and had come for the mouse's removal. I obtained this history from the couple and then reported it to the chief resident on duty, who understandably thought I was fabricating it. Yet the couple stood firm when he questioned them again. Eager to have this nonsense behind him, the resident impatiently "gloved up" and performed a pelvic examination on the woman, only to scream suddenly in pain and withdraw his hand in a flash as a dot of blood began to form under his glove at the tip of a finger. I confess that for a moment I was caught up in the couple's descriptions, wondering how a mouse could actually survive there, lying in wait for any intruder. The chief resident, however, was neither amused nor captured by the mouse metaphor. He was incensed. Calling for more instruments and better lighting, he demolished the mouse metaphor and reduced it to a mechanical one. He found that the woman had a curved surgical needle embedded in the vaginal cuff, the scar at the top of the vagina that is left following a hysterectomy, which she had undergone some years before. Having been lost during surgery, the needle had gradually migrated downward into the vaginal cavity, from which the resident removed it, preventing any further "bites."

My most intense exposure to the pervasive effects of machinelike metaphors for the body came in my first year of medical school while studying anatomy and physiology. *Never* were the endless metaphorical descriptions of the body acknowledged by professors actually to be metaphorical. Could they have assumed that we medical students would automatically know when metaphors—some of which we will examine—were being used? If so, they were wrong. My own hunch is that the professors were as gullible as we. Like us, they had become trapped by their metaphors for the body that alienated us—and our patients—from a comprehensive, integrated view of person and body.

Spouting metaphors at the bedside of a sick patient is a custom highly valued in teaching hospitals, and the patient's bedside is, not surprisingly, one of the main places where young students and physicians learn to think as they do about the body. Students are invariably riveted when an attending physician places his fingers over the femoral artery of a patient he's never seen and barely spoken to, mutters "water hammer pulse," and makes the diagnosis of a leaky aortic valve without ever listening to the heart. Or, equally impressive, the physician may extend and flex the patient's forearm and announce that "cogwheel rigidity" is present and that the correct diagnosis is Parkinson's disease. Students are enchanted by such performances and strive to emulate them. It almost never occurs to students to ask if there might be better metaphors, since most of Western culture—outside medicine as well as within—is enthralled by these machine images. Also, students are presumed to be (and consider themselves to be) in a state of clinical ignorance, and their questioning the appropriateness of body metaphors would be seen by most attending physicians as rank arrogance. Students absorb the metaphors, totally oblivious to the process by which they do. Metaphors accrete gradually, one after the other, like barnacles.

Metaphors are psychologically seductive. They allow the user to convey information with brevity and to appear wise in the process. Unless one realizes this connection to the ego, it is difficult to understand why medical metaphors are such powerful factors in medical education, and why they have such a long and colorful history.

The "snap diagnosis," like the use of medical metaphors, originated in Europe during the eighteenth century, when the mechanical view of the body was in its ascendency. During this period, eminent physicians in the leading medical schools vied with each other in building reputations as shrewd clinicians, just as they compete today as scientists and medical researchers. The trick was to know a diagnosis with as few clues as possible and to communicate it quickly, sometimes theatrically. One of the best snap diagnosticians was Napoleon's favorite physician, Jean-Nicolas Corvisart. He contributed significantly to the art of physical diagnosis and the understanding of cardiac disease. Corvisart added to his reputation by correctly "diagnosing" the subject of an oil painting as a victim of heart disease. So skilled were the well-known physicians Hans von Hebra and Joseph Bell that they could discern not only the diseases of their patients but their occupations as well. The famous German scholar Friedrich Theodor von Frerichs was so infatuated with the cult of snap diagnosis that he never admitted a diagnosis to be wrong. Frerichs was quite dramatic and was worshiped by students, who, it is said, "hung upon his lips, and . . . revered his wonderful precision."[15]

Some physicians see through the pomposity that has always surrounded these customs. I witnessed a superb example of this while assigned to the internal medicine service during my third year in medical school. The attending physician, the faculty member ultimately responsible for the ward, was one of the most renowned cardiologists in the country. In addition to his notoriety as a research cardiologist, he was famous for his expertise at the patient's beside.

During rounds one day we were walking down the hospital corridor when he glanced into a patient's room, held both arms up, and shouted, "STOP!" He came to a sudden halt and stood stark still, completely immobile. We students, interns, and residents who were trailing him—the usual entourage—weren't prepared for the sudden deceleration and bumped into each other like dominoes. Sorting ourselves out, we watched him continue to stare silently at the patient from a distance of about twenty feet, making no effort to enter the room. The object of his fascination was a middle-aged fellow who lay sleeping in bed on a couple of pillows, covered from toes to ears by a white sheet and completely unaware of the physician's presence.

Slowly the attending physician turned to us and announced imperiously, "Severe pump failure. Pistol-shot pulse. Bad aortic valvular insufficiency. Needs his aortic valve replaced now"—a veritable chain of machine metaphors.

Everyone was speechless. We knew the diagnosis was correct because the patient had been admitted earlier that morning, time enough for news about an interesting case to circulate around the ward. But the attending had no way of knowing without being tipped off or having done some extraordinary detective work, which we doubted.

The attending continued to let us stew. He was toying with us and enjoying it. This was Corvisart, Frerichs, and Bell in action at their theatrical, snap-diagnosis best.

Unable to stand the tension, the chief resident eventually spoke up. "But Sir," he said as if taking his cue, "how did you know?"

"It's easy," the attending physician said coolly. "The man is my auto mechanic. I've known about his diagnosis for years!" Then he began to laugh, thoroughly enjoying the joke.

"Look," he went on. "I'm not clairvoyant, and neither are you. Never take shortcuts. There's no substitute for taking a history and performing a physical exam."

We began to chatter with relief. Mastering clinical medicine was hard enough as it was, without the paranormal thrown in.

Although our attending physician exposed the pitfalls of snap diagnosis, he let the machine metaphors for the body stand unchallenged. His example shows that they are alive and well. They are still encountered in studying anatomy, physiology, and pathology in addition to clinical medicine, and a great many of them continue to surface in medical school examinations and in case reports in professional journals. The following list gives only some of the most common metaphors associated with three systems of the body, as well as a few miscellaneous terms. This list may prove enlightening to the layperson, who may not realize just how pervasive the mechanical outlook is.[16]

Cardiovascular System

Water hammer pulse (also known as piston pulse, pistol-shot
    pulse, cannonball pulse)
Machinery murmur
Sawing-wood murmur
Mill-wheel or water-wheel murmur
Bellows murmur
Cannon-shot noise or *bruit de canon*

Nervous System

Cogwheel rigidity
Scissors position
Jackknife epilepsy
[Blitzkrampf or salaam seizure]
Pendular nystagmus
Clasp-knife phenomenon
Hammered skull appearance

Musculoskeletal System

Hammer toe
Mallet finger
Trigger finger
Typewriter finger
Buttonhole rupture
Funnel chest
Screwdriver or Hutchinson's teeth
Silver-fork deformity

Miscellaneous

Sickle-cell disease
Clubbing of the fingers
Hammer and anvil (of the middle ear)
Lockjaw (tetanus)
Sandpaper rash (of scarlet fever)

Although the magnificent clinicians who first constructed these
metaphors had the noblest intentions, they nonetheless contributed to
a vast misunderstanding of how humans function, and set in motion

distorted meanings whose malignant effects continue to reverberate in the lives of patients today. This may sound needlessly contentious to those who believe we've outdistanced the machine metaphor and no longer have a love affair with the gears, levers, pistons, and valves that so infatuated Graves, Corrigan, and their contemporaries. But machinelike meanings still plague us; only the machine's complexity has changed.

A key feature of machines is that they are made of interchangeable parts. They can be disassembled and put back together, like a watch. The parts, moreover, can be removed and sometimes used for other purposes. In keeping with this view, the body has frequently been described in terms of its parts, and what these parts might be good for if removed. Writer Guy Murchie describes how one person saw the body in terms of separate items that could be purchased in a country store. The body, it was said, contained the following:

- water sufficient to fill a ten-gallon keg
- enough fat for seven bars of soap
- enough carbon for 9,000 "lead" pencils
- enough iron to forge a nail
- phosphorous sufficient for 220 matches
- enough magnesium for one dose of "salts"
- enough lime to whitewash a chicken coop
- enough sulfur to purge a dog of fleas[17]

With the disappearance of country stores, linking the body's value to soap, nails, and matches ceased to make much sense. So periodically its worth has been updated to reflect changing times. Murchie reports that about a half-century ago a scientist calculated the body's worth in terms of industrial chemicals and found the total to be about 98 cents. By 1963, however, this figure had risen to $34.54. Writing in 1978, Murchie speculated (with tongue in cheek) that, due to inflation and the increasing scarcity of the elements in the body, the value had quadrupled: we were worth well over $100.

Recently a scientist brought the value of this inventory up to date by comparing it to the cost of purchasing its compounds from chemical companies. He concluded that the body's "market value . . . must be astronomical:"[18]

AMOUNT AND VALUE OF SELECTED CONSTITUENTS OF A 70-KILOGRAM HUMAN BODY

COMPOUND	AMOUNT IN BODY	VALUE
Cholesterol	140 grams	$525.00
Fibrinogen	10.2 grams	$739.50
Hemoglobin	510 grams	$2,550.00
Albumin	153 grams (in serum only)	$4,819.50
Prothrombin	10,200 units	$30,600.00
Immunoglobulin G	34 grams	$30,600.00
Myoglobin	40 grams	$100,000.00

But we are worth even more today; the values above reflect 1983 market prices. And the table doesn't even take into account the value of whole, transplanted organs. Who can put a price on the value of a transplantable heart, two good kidneys, or a pair of fresh corneas? Today we are *so* valuable that it is more tempting than ever to view the body not as just a machine but as a veritable factory. So the value of the body continues to skyrocket, and no one knows what the ceiling may be.

Today steam engines, locks, and dams have been replaced in our fascination with computers. We refer to the "hard wiring," the "neural networks," and the many "programs" and "systems" within the body, and we "store information" and "access memory" in the brain. Although the metaphors have changed, the meaning conveyed is essentially the same: the body, however complicated, is still a machine. As Marvin Minsky, an expert on artificial intelligence at MIT put it, "What is the brain but a computer made of meat?"

MILITARY METAPHORS: THE BODY AT WAR

In addition to being based on machinery, medical metaphors are heavily military in nature. They are linked decisively to the implements and strategies of war, and the metaphors from any given time reflect the *way* the society wages war. The following description of the strategy of medical science dates to 1924, when war was still waged in rather "conventional" ways. In it, land-based, World War I images dominate, and one can almost sense the ebb and flow of trench warfare:

> Until the very recent era . . . medical science has always taken the defensive and has been content to remain dormant until the enemy attacked. To-day, however, medical science has at last become the aggressor, and has penetrated deeply into the disease enemy's terrain.
>
> No longer is mankind content feebly to defend himself against the disease enemy with makeshift weapons and with moss-covered theories and practices. To-day mankind 'foresees the enemy from afar' and takes the aggressive. [The] types of modern weapons [are] too common to call forth comment.[19]

Following the advent of the Cold War, secrecy, stealth, and intrigue crept into the descriptions of bodily events. Not only are we being invaded, the invaders are *foreign* and *invisible*. The pitched battles continue. Consider a description of a stunningly beautiful book of photographs by Lennart Nilsson, one of the most gifted medical photographers of all time (the book's title, *The Body Victorious,* is a clue to what follows):

> Of all the dangers the human body faces during a lifetime— from a broken leg while skiing to a simple papercut—the most prevalent and consistent of these hazards arise from invaders invisible to the naked eye. These are the bacteria, protozoa, fungi and viruses that inhabit our bodies in countless forms and numbers. And it is our own immunological system that strikes with defensive force to rid the body of these foreign cells. . . . This revolutionary photographic essay . . . depicts the architecture of blood clots, the battles between white blood cells and bacteria, killer T-cells attacking cancer and antibodies struggling to locate and repel foreign, sometimes deadly substances in the body, including the AIDS virus.[20]

Metaphors of the body have not failed to keep pace with the space age; one often gets the idea that the field of battle has extended to outer space. An observer recently said of current medical discourse about the immune system:

> A foreign organism invades, perhaps camouflaged as something else. The body, if its advance warning system detects the enemy, puts up a line of defense. Antibodies attack. A lot of killing goes on. Researchers look for magic bullets or guided missiles. The metaphors make it sound as though we each provide a battleground for our own internal Star Wars.[21]

In fact it is the metaphors we use that seem to invade us, like the foreign organisms they purport to describe. And like the bacteria and viruses, when they do they seem to have a life of their own. Metaphors, like microorganisms, actually *move matter*. As we have seen so often in this book, what we *think* about an event—the *meaning* we attribute to it, the *interpretations* we make—translates into actual physical manifestations—changes in heartbeat, respiration, blood pressure, various metabolic pathways, the function of whole organs, even life or death.

MEDICAL STAGES

Another way in which machinelike meanings have crept into medicine can be seen in our penchant for describing medical events in terms of stages or levels. Sophisticated machines are not just on or off; their level of activity can vary. In the same way, sickness can be assigned stages of activity. Almost all cancers are "staged" according to their invasiveness, and heart disease is staged as to its severity. Psychiatrists use Freud's stages of psychosexual development; psychologists employ Piaget's stages of cognitive maturation, Erikson's stages of psychosocial development, Kübler-Ross's stages of death and dying, and the Holmes and Rahe Social Readjustment Rating Scale.

While it can be helpful to think in terms of stages, the habit can get out of hand and become profoundly misleading. We can be tempted to take the stages too literally and think that distinct cutoffs in human existence are being described. This leads us to expect life to be a ratchety, stop-start affair instead of an unbroken, flowing stream of experience. In practice this expectation is manifested in various ways. For example, if the dying person is not progressing through "the right stages" in the predicted order, something is wrong. As medical educator Dr. Howard F. Stein observes, too often the physician may hide behind the metaphor of the "stage" instead of confronting the unique person to whom these terms apply. When this happens, it is the "Stage IV Hodgkins" that gets the attention instead of the patient. The term provides a safety value for physicians: if at a deep psychological level they feel uncomfortable in dealing with their patients, the labels give them some place to hide.[22] But this escape process is employed not just by doctors; it is endemic to our culture:

> Americans don't like tragedy. No matter how complex and heavy a problem, we get our social scientists to give it a name, divide it into stages, and suggest a method for working it through. Then we get our media to publicize the method, and pretty soon there's a 1–800 number to call as an alternative to despair.[23]

In addition—and this may be one of the worst legacies of machinelike metaphors and meanings—when humans are seen as machines it is very difficult for the physician to accept the extraordinary and the unexpected. Machines are deterministic and therefore predictable—one of their essential characteristics is that they "follow the rules." When they "get sick," machines don't experience "miracles," "exceptional cures," or "spontaneous remissions." They don't improve, but only depreciate, break down, wear out, and eventually have to be replaced. Their "clinical course" is always in one direction—toward the junkyard.

But the possibility *always* exists that we will *not* behave like machines when we are sick. This leaves the door open for the occurrence of extraordinary events in *any* human illness—the unexpected cure, the drug that wasn't supposed to work but did, or the illness that "just went away."

The machinelike meanings we attach to our bodies deny that these events are possible. Never has a flat tire or a defunct TV set repaired itself, and neither, these meanings indicate, can our bodies defy the natural order. Cuts may heal and colds may go away, but sooner or later all bodies, like machines, fall apart and die. Bodies, like machines, have certain life expectancies that can be predicted on the basis of how strenuously they are used, whether they contain design flaws (genetic imperfections), and whether they're properly maintained. And in every malady, bodies follow a statistical norm. Thus we hear physicians endlessly addressing patients as if they are machines—reciting dismal "survival" statistics to patients with cancer or heart disease, who "deserve" to know their "chances." Even if the statistics include the remote chance of a cure, the patient seldom hears that part. The meaning that comes through is too often that of doom—a macabre message that all too often is lived out by the patient, who thinks he can't flaunt the physician's prediction and nature's norms. Used in this way, "the numbers" become an inhumane form of communication and an antecedent to death—literally, the "cold" facts.

CAN THE BODY-AS-MACHINE BE A POSITIVE IDEA?

> I am absolutely prepared to talk of the spiritual life of
> an electronic computer; to state that it is reflecting or
> that it is in a bad mood. . . .
>
> —NIELS BOHR[24]

As we saw earlier, the machines that captured the imagination of Graves, Corrigan, and other great figures of early nineteenth-century medicine were simple devices. They followed deterministic physical principles that were well known to scientists of the day. No one believed they possessed minds or were in any sense conscious.

But today, as we've seen, the machines have changed. They are no longer pulleys, levers, or steam engines, but sophisticated, solid state, electronic entities including computers. Many experts in the field of artificial intelligence argue incessantly that certain computers have a mind and are in some sense conscious. To many of these enthusiasts, computers have complex mental lives. They are far more reliable, dispassionate, and less capricious than humans, who seem constitutionally unable to follow the laws of logic for any extended period of time. Some even regard them as morally superior to humans because they are incapable of base motives such as greed, jealously, lust, hatred, and anger. Whether these views are valid is not the point here. What is significant is that for many persons the *meaning* of machines is now different.

In view of this change in the perceived meaning of machines, it is not surprising that the impact on the body of machine metaphors may also be changing. Sometimes the effect of the new machine meanings is highly therapeutic. The following clinical example makes the point:

Michael, a fourteen-year-old boy with newly diagnosed acute leukemia, was being treated with a protracted course of chemotherapy. The nurse assigned to his case, who was responsible for administering the intravenous drugs, discovered that one of his major interests was computers—that, in fact, he was a computer "whiz." As his interest in computers grew, Michael had begun to develop a personal relationship with them. He even named all his components, as if they were pets.

Michael's nurse typically used a form of self-hypnosis during the infusion of the anticancer drugs to lessen discomfort, nausea, and vomiting. The images she employed were those frequently used to facilitate relaxation—visualizing a favorite scene such as a beach or lying peacefully before a warm fire. These were not acceptable to Michael. He implored the nurse to let him invent his own mental imagery, and she agreed.

In his imagination Michael would transform himself into his favorite computer and assume its emotional qualities, which for him were real. This included absolute tranquillity and reliability. In this state, his body could perform the most difficult functions with the greatest of ease and at enormous speed. He visualized his body as an immensely intelligent "program" that was fully capable of integrating the potent drugs and dispatching them to the cancer cells where they would do their work with perfect effectiveness. He reasoned that, since computers never get nauseated, neither would he. At the end of each chemotherapy session he would "save" and "store" what his body had learned, which he would "open" and activate when the next treatment session began.

Michael experienced a complete remission from his acute leukemia and, years later, is disease free.

During the course of his chemotherapy, his nurse asked him what it meant to him to be a computer.

"It means being powerful," he replied. "It makes me feel strong and wise. I don't have to do everything myself—it's already in the program. I know everything is going to come out O.K., because my computer is smarter than I am and it can think faster, too. Besides, it's fun!"[25]

The effect of the mechanical metaphors on Michael's body did not depend on whether they were true in some absolute sense, but on whether they were true *for him*. Using his own unique metaphors, he created a *meaning* of his body, which helped him activate the innate healing potential contained in all human bodies. He intuitively recognized the body for what it is—an awesomely effective survival machine containing the accumulated wisdom of several million years. Michael gave himself over to this vast reservoir of biological wisdom, which he conceived as his own inner "program." His basic strategy involved trust—cooperating with the power that was already there, not generating it himself.

When we try to predict how the meaning of a metaphor will affect patients we must always bear in mind the invividualistic, idiosyncratic nature of metaphors. The same metaphor or image may work differently on each person. What if Michael had been a fifty-year-old employee of an insurance company who couldn't make the switch to computers and had just been bypassed for promotion, fired, or given early "retirement"? For him, "computer" would carry a totally different meaning, which would undoubtedly lead to a different body response if he tried to use the image in any sort of treatment. For him, the very thought of computers might *generate* nausea, not prevent it. This means that those health care professionals using metaphorical and imagistic techniques therapeutically must be skillful and artistic, since the effects are not predictable.

This point needs emphasizing. As great numbers of people have discovered the effect of mind on body, an intense search has developed for a formula—the "right" images or the "best" thoughts to employ in any given situation. Many "authorities" actually advocate a backward readout process, in which one can look up in a chart or table a specific symptom or body part that is problematic, correlate this with the actual thought or constellation of emotions that led to it, and then employ certain psychological measures to counteract the disease-causing emotions. If the symptom is AIDS, for example, the causative feelings that made one susceptible are frequently said to be "rejection of one's true identity" or "inability to accept who one really is," and the therapeutic thoughts prescribed are positive affirmations about personal identity and self-esteem. This approach implies that AIDS signifies a similarity in the psyche of all who contract it, a nonsensical implication, especially considering the broad spectrum of people who contract AIDS—homosexuals, prostitutes, addicts, hemophiliacs, "straight" wives of profligate or bisexual men, surgeons, and unborn babies. The shallowness of this formulaic approach has been emphasized by Doctors Joan and Myrin Borysenko in their seminars. "Imagine a huge black dog," they say. "One person might respond to this image with horror and fear, another by wanting to rush up to the dog to hug, kiss, and wrestle with it—all depending on their previous experiences with pets."

"Black dog"—like all meanings—is inconstant. This point was consistently emphasized by the Swiss psychologist C. G. Jung in his interpretation of dreams. Jung decried assigning fixed meanings to dreams. Ultimately they derive their meaning *only* in the context of an individual person's experience.

Fixing meanings to various thoughts and images is in my opinion misleading and inhumane. It totally misconstrues the way meaning operates. It assumes that images, thoughts, meanings, and metaphors affect everyone identically just because their surface content is the same. Unfortunately this idea *reinforces* a picture of humans as machines, because it conceives of them as entities who respond identically to any given input. Most persons perpetrating this view are well-meaning individuals who want only the best for their clients or patients. Yet their disguised, machinelike perspectives can paradoxically do great harm by minimizing, not maximizing, the power of consciousness to aid in health.

Tolerance, artistry, and sophistication are required in the use of all "meaning therapies." What if Michael's nurse had responded negatively to his picture of himself as a complicated machine, whether because of her negative experiences with this image in other cancer patients or because she did not think of herself as a computer? In this case, Michael would have been denied a powerful assist in his healing.

Will the meanings of machines for our culture continue to evolve, so that future generations can use them as positively as Michael? Or will machine metaphors continue to weigh us down with their predominantly negative implications? We cannot be sure. What we *can* be certain of, however, is that the effect of metaphors on the body will never be absolute, but will vary according to the meaning they contain for each person. This means that no single metaphor should ever command our categorical endorsement *or* condemnation—including the metaphor of the body as machine.

In spite of the fact that machine metaphors might take the form of more human meanings as in Michael's case, we nonetheless should realize their innate limitations. Although computers *are* more complex than steam engines or any of the other machines to which humans have compared themselves in the past, we should not wish to instate *any* machine no matter how complex, as the standard against which we compare ourselves. The reason is that machine models seem always to leave out the qualities that make us quintessentially human. This is expressed by psychologist Lawrence LeShan in his important book *The Dilemma of Psychology:*

Conceivably . . . a computer could be designed that could write acceptable poetry. But there is not the possibility of a computer that, after encoding and recording a poem, would actively desire to buy a bunch of flowers for another computer and to live with it forever. Or a computer that could experience awe in a cathedral or that, falling apart of old age, would wish deeply for the comforting presence of its mother.[26]

THE TOMATO EFFECT

By dominating our views of the body and how illness originates, metaphors also dominate the treatments and therapies that are available to us. If we see the body as a machine, we seek out therapies that are mechanical, as we have now done for the better part of three hundred years.

An example of this occurred when DMSO (dimethyl sulfoxide), a commercial solvent, became popular a few years ago as a treatment for various forms of arthritis. Applied directly to the skin over the joints, DMSO seemed to have remarkable powers of penetration, and arthritis patients began to swear by it. Many described the use of DMSO in machinelike terms. They were "lubricating" themselves, just as they might lubricate the chassis of their car. A patient of mine even switched to WD-40, a popular commercial lubricant that "takes the squeaks out," and was confident it was superior. He would spray his joints with the aerosol can just as he sprayed his door hinges or the wheels of his lawn mower. The use of machine lubricants in medicine is hardly new. A century ago one of the most popular household remedies in rural America was the lubricant of the day: axle grease.

If we encounter therapies that do not fit our preconceived ideas about what an appropriate treatment should be, we may reject them *even if evidence for their effectiveness is staring us in the face*—a response that researchers James S. and Jean M. Goodwin have called the "tomato effect."

The origin of this term is rooted in historical fact. When the tomato (*Lycopersicon esculentum*) was discovered in the New World, it was carried back to Spain from whence it rapidly spread to Italy, where it was called *pomodoro,* and to France. The French called it *pomme d'amour,* believing it to have aphrodisiac properties. By 1560 the tomato was well on its way to becoming a staple in the European diet.

Although this exotic South American fruit was revolutionizing European eating habits (along with other New World discoveries such as corn, potatoes, beans, cacao, and tobacco), in North America it was ignored or actively shunned.[27] The tomato was not even cultivated in North America during the 1700s, and not until the 1800s did North Americans regard it as edible. Commercial cultivation remained rare until the twentieth century, although today the tomato had been called our largest commercial food crop.

The tomato was reviled in North America because people "knew" it was poisonous. After all, it belongs to the "deadly nightshade" family (Solanaceae). The leaves and fruits of several members of this family, including belladonna and mandrake, can cause death if eaten in sufficient quantity. As Goodwin and Goodwin point out, "The fact that the French and Italians were eating tomatoes in increasing quantities without seeming harm did not encourage colonial Americans to try them. It simply did not make sense to eat poisonous food. Not until 1820, when Robert Gibbon Johnson ate a tomato on the steps of the courthouse in Salem, New Jersey, and survived, did the people of America begin, grudgingly, we suspect, to consume tomatoes."[28]

Throughout history we have been blind to effective therapies that did not "make sense" and we have ignored positive changes in illness when they were used—the tomato effect in action. The use of colchicine, one of the most efficacious medications ever discovered, is a classic example of how preconceived meanings can hide the truth. The use of colchicine (derived from the crocuslike colchicum plant) to treat gout, one of humankind's most painful afflictions, dates back to the fifth century, and knowledgeable therapists used it thereafter for a thousand years. But after the thirteenth century all mention of colchicine as a treatment for gout disappeared from medical writings. It was not introduced into the West again until 1780, when it again became recognized as one of the most effective medications known to man. How could it have disappeared for four hundred years? As Copeman explained, "This is a strange page in medical history. . . . [With] the Renaissance [came] the dominance of scholars who, with all this written and practical evidence before them chose to see none of it—their learning seemed like a bandage round their eyes."[29] The major problem was that colchicum and other *specific* treatments ceased to make sense. With the Renaissance came a return to the medical teachings and practices of Galen and Hippocrates. To them, all disease resulted from a nonspecific imbalance of bodily constituents. Specific cures for specific illnesses, then, while perfectly reasonable for the medieval mind steeped in religion and magic, were repugnant to the enlightened physicians of the Renaissance, who preferred the classical therapies for gout, such as bleeding and purging.[30]

The use of high-dose aspirin in the treatment of rheumatoid arthritis is another classic example of the tomato effect. Extracts of the bark of the willow tree are a natural source of aspirin and have been used off and on for three thousand years to treat pain and fever. When aspirin was synthesized and produced commercially in the late 1800s, high-dose aspirin therapy became the treatment of choice for acute rheumatic fever, and by the end of the nineteenth century it was also recognized as an effective treatment for rheumatoid arthritis. But at the same time, the theory that rheumatoid arthritis was caused by an infectious agent was on the rise. In view of this theory, it simply made no sense to think that aspirin, which helped pain and fever, could be of any use in rheumatoid arthritis. Thus clinicians became blind to the fact that it was an effective treatment—all because the *meaning* of the disease for them changed. Thus, from 1900 to 1950, every major medical textbook and every article on the treatment of rheumatoid arthritis either did not mention aspirin or made brief mention that low doses given intermittently might help the pain. By the early 1950s the meaning of the disease had changed again: the infectious theory of the origin of the illness was discarded, and it came to be viewed as due to chronic inflammation of unknown origin. During this same period, studies in animals showed aspirin capable of relieving inflammation in addition to calming fever and pain. Thus, in the mid-1950s, most textbooks and review articles again took up the theme that had lain dormant for a half-century: aspirin in high doses was an effective treatment for rheumatoid arthritis.[31]

Some of the current "tomatoes" exist because of the hypnotic power of our mechanical conceptions of the body. Machines aren't conscious, we say, and cannot think. Treatments for them, therefore, must also be mindless—for example, scalpels (the wrench or hammer), transplants or genetically redesigned cells (replacement parts), and drugs (the lubricants). This means that any therapy relying on the ability of the mind to affect the body is likely to go unnoticed.

A prime example is the treatment of coronary artery disease, the most common cause of death in our society. We pursue with a passion the elimination of major *physical* factors—smoking, high blood pressure, high blood cholesterol, and diabetes mellitus—although most people who have their first heart attack have *none* of these risk factors present.[32] As we have seen, evidence suggests that the most important risk factor for the development of heart attack is something decidely mental—*job dissatisfaction*.[33] This finding had been strengthened by the discovery that more fatal heart attacks occur on Monday than on any other day, and that they cluster around 9:00 A.M., the beginning of the workweek (the Black Monday syndrome, see page 62). This is a remarkably odd finding, since, as far as we know, no other mammals die more frequently on a particular day of the week. The tomato? Studies have also affirmed that attention to emotional factors such as overall fulfillment and satisfaction in persons who have had heart attacks can reduce the rate of subsequent heart attacks and death.[34] Yet this therapy continues, for the most part, to be ignored as if it did not exist—the tomato effect in action. Almost all our efforts go into mechanical therapies such as coronary artery bypass surgery—sometimes called an *emotional* bypass—and the use of cardiac drugs. Why? Mainly because the entire process of arteriosclerosis and coronary artery disease is believed to be a mindless, mechanical process requiring mechanical—not mental—interventions.

Cancer therapy, like treatment for heart disease, is a veritable tomato patch, and for the same reason: like heart disease, cancer has been viewed solely as a mechanical process requiring physical interventions. For more than a decade, studies suggesting that mental and emotional factors are important in the development and survival of cancer have for the most part been ignored or actually shouted down. The dominant message, incessantly preached from the editorial pages of medical journals and the podiums of medical schools, is that the "inherent biology of the disease" is overwhelmingly important and that feelings, emotions, and attitudes are simply along for the ride.

Professor David Spiegel, a psychiatrist and researcher at Stanford University Medical School, set out to refute the idea that mental factors were important in the course of diseases. Like many clinicians, he felt that assigning a role to the mind in cancer was not only erroneous but potentially destructive as well. (Many believe this idea generates guilt on the part of the cancer patient because it suggests that he or she was somehow responsible for causing the disease.)

Spiegel followed eighty-six women with breast cancer for a period of ten years. Those who received group therapy and lessons in self-hypnosis lived an average of *twice as long* as those who were given only traditional medical treatment. Spiegel described himself as "stunned" at this finding, which contradicted his expectations.[35]

Yet his results are not unique. Other researchers have demonstrated similar findings in recent years, only to be "tomatoed"—ignored for the most part by clinicians and by federal and foundational funding sources. Others, such as pioneers Carl and Stephanie Simonton, who a decade ago demonstrated a doubling of survival in cancer patients using imagery and visualization techniques, were tomatoed in the worst possible way. They were officially condemned by the American Cancer Society as employing "unproved methods"—an action akin to the excommunication of heretics.[36] But just as official attitudes toward the use of gout and aspirin shifted, so, too, the orthodox attitude toward the role of the mind in cancer is changing. Today Stephanie Simonton is actively pursuing her research in a major medical school, and Carl Simonton's early predictions are gaining wider acceptance through solid scientific work such as Spiegel's.

Goodwin and Goodwin point out many other tomatoes that currently exist. Perhaps the main lesson from the tomato effect is this: *There is no monolithic, external, objective set of facts to which we can appeal in determining what is medically real; our medical reality, including the therapies we deem to be valuable, is deeply affected by the meanings we glean, which are in turn guided by the metaphors we employ. Meanings and metaphors are powerful determinants not only of what we observe, but of what we can observe.*

THE SNAKEROOT EFFECT

One of the most mysterious diseases to appear on the American frontier was "milk sickness."[37] Like the black plague which decimated medieval Europe, this illness carried away whole segments of rural communities. Ecologist David Cameron Duffy, on whose work the following description is based, estimates that in a single year milk sickness killed one-tenth of the population of Danville, Indiana, one-fourth the population of Madison County, Ohio, and as many as half the people in Dubois County, Indiana. Children were the most susceptible, but no group was spared. Perhaps the most famous victim was Nancy Hanks Lincoln, Abraham Lincoln's mother, who died in Little Pigeon Creek, Illinois.

A patient with milk sickness demonstrated a constellation of symptoms—extreme weakness, nausea, thirst, constipation, and a burning sensation in the stomach. The breath smelled foul like turpentine, which skilled physicians regarded as a valuable clue to the disease's identity. Fever was usually absent, separating this disease from typhoid fever and other infections. Death usually came in two to ten days. Sometimes the patient would appear to recover, then relapse and die. In those who did not succumb, symptoms sometimes lingered for months or years.

By 1810, milk sickness was recognized as a separate, distinct disease. Theories focused on the fact that it was rare in populated areas while striking the pioneers who carved farms out of the forests beyond the Appalachians. Some doctors thought it was caused by a microorganism in the soil. Others thought it was a poisoning of some sort—possibly due to bad water, to spiders or flies, to certain plants or mushrooms, to metals such as arsenic, lead, copper, or cobalt, or to noxious gases from decaying vegetation.

Early on, settlers recognized that milk sickness occurred in areas where cattle suffered from a disease known as trembles. This scourge manifested as slow movement, foul breath, profound trembling after slight exertion, and lying down to die. The cattle that died seemed to be those grazing on rich woodland pastures. Humans who drank milk or ate meat from them frequently developed milk sickness. This connection was so obvious to pioneers in Tennessee that in 1821 the state legislature passed a law requiring fencing to be built around certain forested areas "to prevent animals from eating an unknown vegetable, thereby imparting to their milk and flesh qualities highly deleterious."

The primary suspects among the "unknown vegetables" were poison ivy and white snakeroot. There were problems with the poison ivy hypothesis. For one thing, poison ivy did not grow well in deep forests, which was where cattle seemed to contract the disease. Moreover, when forests were cut and the soil cultivated, which were the best ways to exterminate milk sickness, poison ivy would sometimes grow more vigorously. There were also problems with the white snakeroot explanation, as this plant grew quite well in many places where milk sickness was rare.

The earliest noteworthy experiments on the frontier were made by Anna Pierce, an enterprising woman who was schooled as a nurse and midwife and who settled in Illinois as as physician. Around 1828, milk sickness swept through Pierce's family, killing her mother and sister-in-law and leaving her father seriously weakened. In the wake of this devastation, she made several important observations about milk sickness and trembles—milk sickness often came from drinking milk; it was worse during the growing season; lactating cows were usually spared; and horses, which ate more grass than herbs, were relatively unaffected, suggesting that some broad-leafed, herbaceous plant was the culprit. Pierce thus urged people in her area to abstain from drinking milk from June until the first frosts of autumn. And what about the identity of the poisonous plant? A Shawnee woman, who was a fugitive from the forced resettlement of her people and who was known only as Aunt Shawnee, took Pierce to the woods and showed her the white snakeroot plant. She told Pierce that the white snakeroot plant was indeed the cause of both trembles and milk sickness. Pierce fed snakeroot to a calf; it developed trembles. Convinced by her experiments, Pierce then started a program for the local eradication of the plant. She grew some in her garden and invited neighboring physicians to view it, so they could identify it and promote extermination efforts in their own areas.

Other observers confirmed the toxic nature of snakeroot. Several years after Pierce's experiments, an Ohio farmer named John Roe fed the plant to a steer and to a cow that was nursing a calf. The steer was dead in seven days, the calf in nine. In the 1880s, various physicians, farmers, and scientists repeated and validated Roe's experiment.

In spite of consistent findings that snakeroot was highly toxic, some authorities discounted the idea as nonsense. They preferred to focus on noxious gases and metal poisoning. Incredibly, other doctors refused even to believe the disease existed, dismissing it as "a mere matter of credulous fancy." Some people went to great lengths to disprove the snakeroot hypothesis. One disbeliever chewed the plant to prove its safety; he suffered for a month before finally dying. In another challenge of snakeroot's toxicity, a disbeliever (a doctor) furnished a calf, while a believer (a farmer) furnished the snakeroot. As in the previous experiments, the animal died.

In 1905 definitive experiments were done by Dr. Edwin Mosely, who fed snakeroot to a variety of animals—mice, rabbits, dogs, and sheep—and determined the dosage required for fatality. He found that snakeroot is less poisonous in wet years than in dry years and that it remains poisonous even after being killed by frosts. Others found that snakeroot varies regionally in potency, being weakest in the east and south and strongest in the west. In 1928, Dr. James Couch isolated a chemical called tremetol from snakeroot, injected it into animals, and showed that it caused trembles. At Stanford University in the 1960s, chemists demonstrated that tremetol is comprised of several chemicals, the most common of which, tremetone, is similar to rotenone, an insecticide highly toxic to fish. And in 1987, other researchers found that the chemicals in snakeroot are not themselves poisonous until converted metabolically in the body to other compounds.

Even after Mosely's 1905 experiments, the evidence was still resisted strongly. Dr. Crawford of the U.S. Department of Agriculture for example, remained a major skeptic. In an experiment of his own, he fed snakeroot to six rabbits. Three of the rabbits died, and two others developed trembles. Yet Crawford still *continued to believe snakeroot safe*! Crawford thus performed the ultimate experiment: he ate snakeroot himself. He survived, because it was the relatively safe eastern form of the plant he ingested.

The "snakeroot effect" is the refusal to acknowledge that a treatment or substance is *harmful* in spite of overwhelming evidence. As such, it is the opposite of the tomato effect, the refusal to acknowledge that a treatment or substance is *helpful*. And like the tomato effect, it is pervasive in our culture, affecting both laypersons and professionals.

The history of medicines in the United States is full of "snakeroots." Phenacetin was once widely used in headache remedies. Even when phenacetin was convincingly shown to cause kidney damage and was removed from the market, many people continued to swear by its effectiveness as a headache medication and continued to use it.

When tryptophan, an amino acid widely used to promote sleep, was recently taken off the market because of its association with the sometimes fatal "eosinophilia-myalgia" syndrome, a black market developed to supply those insomniacs who remained loyal.

Scientifically trained physicians can be especially susceptible to the snakeroot effect. When a treatment appears as if it *should* work—when it *seems* rational and logical—it is likely to continue to be used even after scientific studies have shown it harmful. An example is the use of anticoagulants or "blood thinning" medications for patients suspected of an impending heart attack. When their use was proposed by Patrick Mounsey in 1951, it was thought that an actual clot in a coronary artery—a coronary thrombosis—preceded a heart attack and that this could be prevented by administrating medications that prevented clotting.[38] Although this seemed completely rational, evidence against these medications accumulated and prompted a noted authority on heart disease to state, "there is no evidence that these drugs alter the incidence of [myocardial] infarction or the natural history of [this] illness."[39] Moreover, there was substantial evidence that anticoagulants were harmful and dangerous, in some cases causing death from internal bleeding. In spite of this, many physicians continued to use them as if they actually were beneficial—the snakeroot effect in action.

Another snakeroot that died hard was the habit of prolonged bed rest and relative immobility for patients following heart attack. Long after these three- and four-week periods of convalescence were shown to cause complications such as thrombophlebitis and pulmonary emboli (clots in the veins and lungs), and much shorter periods of rehabilitation were proved to be safer and more effective, the old practice retained its popularity.

Surgery is a veritable graveyard of snakeroots. Many types of operations have through the years been greeted with wild enthusiasm, later to be discredited as worthless and even harmful, only to continue to be valued by some physicians in spite of the incriminating evidence. Radical mastectomy for breast cancer; the "stomach stapling procedure" for massive obesity, in which the size of the stomach is made smaller; and various procedures to relieve angina pectoris and prevent heart attacks are examples.

Whether we refuse to acknowledge harmful therapies or to

believe in helpful ones, the reason is often the same: our images of the body exert powerful effects on us and largely determine what we consider rational. These images are almost always of a mechanical nature and affect not only what we observe but what we *can* observe. They put themselves between us and therapies that are nonmechanical in nature, many of which are discussed in Part III, "Healing Breakthroughs."

Nonmechanical images of the body and treatments based on them are not, however, a perfect solution for self-deception; they do not guarantee that we will more quickly accept potent treatments and reject harmful ones. Plenty of tomatoes and snakeroots exist in nonmechanical approaches to the body as well as in mechanical ones. But being open to nonmechanical images of the body *does* mean that we have more therapeutic options to choose from, more pieces of the puzzle to work with. Healing, as a result, can become less remote, cold, and mechanistic—and more effective, humane, and fulfilling for both patient and therapist.

"In tribal societies," Ean Begg states "when meaning grew cold and the waters of life ceased to flow, the chief or shaman would sometimes have a big dream which could result in the establishment of a new dance or religious ritual of great importance for the psychological well-being of the tribe, which would thereby once again feel linked to the source of meaning and life." If we are to shed our defeating, stifling beliefs about the body—that it is mindless, material, doomed, and meaningless—we need a new dream of the body, some new image that can help us restore new life and hope.

Today many new images are arising. The next chapter presents one such image, consistent with modern science and linked also to many "big dreams" of the past: the image of the body as *music*.

The Body as Music

> If the arrangement of the whole (universe) is some
> kind of a musical harmony . . . in human nature, the
> whole music of the universe can be discerned. . . .
>
> —GREGORY OF NYSSA
> (ca. A.D. 330–395)[1]

Many living organisms communicate so richly through sound that it is hard to imagine their survival without it. In many species the life-sustaining processes of mating and reproduction rely solidly on systems of calls—bird song and the songs of whales are examples—which are bewilderingly complex and in some cases decidedly musical. Sound and the continuation of life go hand in hand.

In humans, the physical body reflects the sound we perceive, down to the biochemical level. So sensitive are we to sound that noise pollution has been called the most common modern health hazard. High levels of unpleasant sounds cause blood vessels to constrict; increase the blood pressure, pulse, and respiratory rates; release extra fats into the bloodstream; and cause the blood's magnesium level to fall. Noxious sounds are a hazard in the modern hospital, where there can be a steady barrage of sonic unpleasantness. Patients recovering from heart attacks in coronary care units are particularly susceptible to unpleasant sounds; noise pollution in these settings can affect survival and recovery.[2]

People are disturbed not only by loud sounds but also by sounds that are dissonant or inharmonic. They can also be disturbed by silence. If healthy persons are confined to bed and exposed to soft but varied harmonic sounds, they perceive their environment more restful than do subjects who are in a completely quiet environment.[3]

But sounds can mean something to us that is not adequately explained by an analysis of the physical changes they cause. Some are tied to levels of reality beyond the physical processes of mating, reproduction, species survival, and bodily chemistry. Larry Ephron of Berkeley, California, has suggested that certain sounds are connected to the recognition of transcendent and spiritual realities. The repetition of these sounds conveys something that cannot be analyzed in terms of decibels or cycles per second. As he says,

> It suddenly came to me . . . that the word for the spirit of the universe or whatever you want to call "It" has the sound "aahhh" in many languages. To wit: God, Jahı, Ra, Allah, Brahma, Atman, Yahweh, Ram, Baal, Ahura Mazda (I'm using the thesaurus), Og, Hachiman, Mab, nagual, mana, wakan, huaca. . . . I think it's because the "aahhh" sound is so relaxing of the jaw and throat, letting go, giving in to what is. Makes me reminded of the oneness of all us folks.[4]

For millennia, many great spiritual traditions have prescribed the repetition of certain sounds that are known to promote the experience of transcendent realities. The ritualistic use of specific chants, prayers, incantations, affirmations, and holy words is truly worldwide. Are these sounds affecting our spiritual health, just as other sounds can affect our physical health? Could certain sounds affect *both* our physical and spiritual well-being—a kind of sonic wonder drug that works on all the dimensions of human experience? There is evidence for this possibility. Certain meditation practices that emphasize the repetitious chanting of special sounds, or mantras, are associated with demonstrable health benefits. For example, Transcendental Meditation (TM), which employs mantras, has been helpful in treating serious medical problems such as irregular heart rhythms,[5] and evidence suggests that the prolonged use of TM can reverse many aspects of the aging process. Statistics also show that the rate of hospital admissions and the overall health costs of TM practitioners are lower than those of nonmeditators.[6]

Although we ordinarily think silence excludes sound, certain sounds can be helpful, paradoxically, in coming to the Great Silence of which all the major spiritual traditions speak. This is the mystical experience of oneness and unity of all things, that state of emptiness where the recognition of a higher reality can take place.

Cultivation of *silence* has also been shown to have positive health benefits. In one study, when men with high blood cholesterol levels learned to quiet their mental activity for twenty minutes twice a day while simply sitting in a chair, their cholesterol levels fell by one-third.[7]

As we shall now see, sounds—particularly music—can open the possibility for an entirely new meaning of the body, a counter to the mechanical views that have recently dominated our thinking.

IS DNA MUSICAL?—THE BODY AS A MELODY

> Music is a strange thing. I would almost say it is a miracle. For it stands half way between thought and phenomenon, between spirit and matter, a sort of nebulous mediator, like and unlike each of the things it mediates—spirit that requires manifestation in time and matter that can do without space . . . we do not know what music is.
>
> —HEINRICH HEINE[8]

Why are we moved by music? One reason may be that the body itself is intrinsically musical, right down to the DNA that makes up our genes.

The idea that DNA and music might be connected comes from the work of Dr. Susumu Ohno, a geneticist at the Beckman Research Institute of the City of Hope in Duarte, California.[9] The genes of every organism are composed of strands of DNA, which in turn are made up of four nucleotides containing the bases adenine, guanine, cytosine, and thymine, arranged in sequences that are unique for each species. In an imaginative leap, Dr. Ohno assigned musical notes to these substances—*do* to cytosine, *re* and *mi* to adenine, *fa* and *sol* to guanine, and *la* and *ti* to thymine. Then, having assigned musical notes to each base, Dr. Ohno chose a particular key and timing, as well as the duration of each note. The result was a melodic composition that was finally fleshed out with harmonies by his wife, Midori, a musician. When completely transcribed, the scores were then performed by professional musicians on instruments such as the piano or organ, violin, and viola.

Dr. Ohno has notated over fifteen songs of the DNA of a variety of living organisms during the past two years. He finds that the more evolved an organism is, the more complicated is the music. The DNA of a single-cell protozoan, for example, translates into a simple four-note repetition. But the music transcribed from human DNA from, e.g., the body's receptor site for insulin is much more complex. Listeners knowledgeable about music have taken these DNA-based compositions for the music of Bach, Brahms, Chopin, and other great composers. These melodies are majestic and inspiring. Many persons hearing them for the first time are moved to tears; they cannot believe their bodies, which they believed to be mere collections of chemicals, contain such uplifting, inspiring harmonies—that they are *musical*.

Not only is it possible to make music starting with DNA, but one can also do the reverse—start with great pieces of music, assign nucleotides to the notes, and end up with a particular type of DNA. When Dr. Ohno transcribed a Chopin piece into a chemical notation, sections of the resulting formula were the DNA of a human cancer gene. It seems that even cancers have their own music![10]

Many great artists, writers, and musicians have heard messages in nature, some of them musical. When Mozart heard a complex, lengthy piece of music fully formed, where was it coming from? When Hesse said in the prologue to *Demian* that he had learned to listen to the messages his blood whispers to him, what was he actually hearing? How do we explain synesthetes, those individuals whose senses operate together in such a way that they can smell sounds and see musical tones? Where is this information coming from? Are they in touch with some music encoded in their bodies?

Concert pianist Lorin Hollander has described the rich visual imagery he has experienced all his life on playing the works of the great composers. These images, he states, often take the form of highly complex geometric designs. His experience affirms Pythagoras's assertion in the sixth century B.C.: "There is geometry in the humming of the strings. There is music in the spacings of the spheres." Hollander was astonished when he later discovered that these forms, which he had visualized since childhood, were practically identical to many of the beautiful tile designs of Islamic mosques scattered throughout the Middle East and India. The pentagonal and hexagonal shapes that are repeated in these designs show striking similarity to the way DNA is represented in two-dimensional chemical notation. In the body the nucleotides that make up DNA are not, of course, two-dimensional figures; that is only the way we draw them "on paper." But that may be the way they display themselves to the imagination—whether to Hollander, whose music calls them forth, to molecular biologists, or to the great artists who embellished the mosques of Islam.

If connecting DNA and music seems fanciful, we should recall that there is no reason in principle why DNA has to be described in the familiar alphabetical symbols of organic chemistry—C for carbon, N for nitrogen, O for oxygen, H for hydrogen, and so forth. It could be described using many symbols, even musical notes. If we were imaginative enough to think musically as well as alphabetically, this just might permit us to hear the music of the body. This experience could provide us with nobler visions of the body, and might allow us at long last to escape the tyranny of machine thinking.

Recognizing the music latent in DNA suggests a new way of looking at evolution. Rather than a method of passing *genes* from one generation to another, the evolutionary process could be a way of passing the *music* along, each generation "making music" for the next. Mutations would be ways of tinkering with the melody, of creating new, more complex tunes. "Survival of the fittest" might mean "staying in key," "playing with the orchestra," or "maintaining the harmony." The natural world would not be "nature red in tooth and claw," it would be a gigantic symphony instead, composed of innumerable instruments. Since some structures in humans are the same as in distant species like protozoa and mice—the chemical receptors for insulin and endorphins are examples—we might conceive of ourselves as "in the same section of the orchestra" as these species, or as "playing the same instrument." Instead of sitting imperiously atop the evolutionary chain, we might see ourselves as simply occupying the "first chair," dependent on our "colleagues" to flesh out the score and enrich the performance. We might even begin to think of the Absolute not as a blind watchmaker who fashioned a mindless machine, but as the Maestro who wrote the melody and interwove all the harmonies.

But the material world is more than just the DNA of living creatures; it is nonliving things such as rocks, stars, and galaxies as well. One could conceivably notate *any* of these things musically. When Pythagoras spoke in the sixth century B.C. of "the music of the spheres," was he comprehending this sort of notation in the heavens? Could the music in our genes reflect the music of the universe? After all, the stuff of which our bodies are made was spawned in remote galaxies, and the atomic components of our DNA have been processed through the lifetimes of several stars. Is the vast universe, then, the source of the primordial melodies that eventually precipitated in our protoplasm? Is the cosmos an immense music bank from which the music of our DNA is on loan? Was Plotinus correct when he said, "All music, based upon melody and rhythm, is the earthly representative of heavenly music"?

Many of the scientists who have pondered the nature of the universe have responded deeply to music. Pythagoras measured harmonies on a lyre string; Nobel physicist Richard Feynman beat salsa rhythms on his bongos; and Nobelist in physical chemistry Ilya Prigogine is a gifted pianist. Lawrence LeShan has noted that at the famous Copenhagen Conference of 1932, which was attended by the greatest physicists of the day, there was enough musical talent and training for a first-rate orchestra.[11] The thoughts of Einstein, who was famous for his affection for the violin, come tantalizingly close to uniting the scientific and musical visions. He said, "[Music and scientific research] are nourished by the same source of longing, and they complement one another in the release they offer."[12]

Plotinus's suggestion of a music-permeated cosmos echoes through many traditions. The legendary Zen patriarch Lao-tzu spoke of the Great Tone that is "the tone that goes beyond all usual imagination." In the Hindu tradition the Great Tone is *Nada Brahma,* the tone from which God made the world, "which continues to sound at the bottom of creation, and which sounds through everything."[13]

The image is one of music embedded in everything, perhaps in human tissue itself. Could different body parts "have their own music," music that is more differentiated than the DNA music shared by all cells as suggested by Professor Ohno? Could they *respond* to certain music?

Without doubt, body parts can respond to the "wrong" music. The British neurologist Macdonald Critchley cites examples from long ago: in 1605, LeLoirier's *Treatise of Spectres* told of an individual who experienced urinary incontinence on hearing the music of the lyre, and Shakespeare in *The Merchant of Venice* spoke of "some that are mad if they behold a cat, and others when the bagpipe sing i'th'nose cannot contain their urine." Critchley relates a famous case dating to 1913 in St. Petersburg of a rare disease known as musicogenic epilepsy—epilepsy brought on by music. It involved, ironically, the well-known music critic Nikonov. His first attack came when he was at the Imperial Opera House watching a performance of Meyerbeer's *The Prophet.* During the third act he became tremulous and sweaty and his left eye began to twitch uncontrollably. He developed a severe headache and lost consciousness. Nikonov thereafter became a prey to these attacks, each brought on by music and nothing else. Even at a distance, music would trigger epilepsy. As a result, he was tormented by a veritable phobia of hearing music. "If out of doors the sound of an approaching military band reached him, he would stop his ears, and seek refuge in a back street or any handy doorway or shop." Eventually the attacks became more or less controlled with medication.[14]

In contrast, could certain tissues become healthier if "their music" were played? Perhaps. Many healers throughout history have realized the body's capacity to respond to certain music. In 1529, Caelius Aurelianus wrote of a musician who could literally make specific parts of the body dance: "A certain piper would play his instrument over the affected parts and these would begin to throb and palpitate, banishing the pain and bringing relief."[15] And Aulus Gellius, writing circa A.D. 160, said,

I ran across the statement very recently in the book of Theophrastus *On Inspiration* that many men have believed and put their belief on record, that when gouty pains in the hips are most severe they are relieved if a fluteplayer plays soothing measures. That snake-bites are cured by the music of the flute, when played skillfully and melodiously, is also stated in a book of Democritus, entitled *On Deadly Infections,* in which he shows that the music of the flute is medicine for many ills that flesh is heir to. So very close is the connection between the bodies and the minds of men, and therefore, between physical and mental ailments and their remedies.

It is not just in the stories of antiquity that we see the healing power of music. A child psychologist recently reported his experience with an eleven-year-old boy who was diagnosed as a catatonic schizophrenic. The child had not uttered a word in seven years. In one session with him, the therapist played Bach's *Jesu, Joy of Man's Desiring.* The boy began to weep. When the music ended he announced through his tears, "That is the most powerful music I have ever heard; now I can speak!"[16]

If the body can respond so decisively to music, it must in some sense *be* music. As Goethe put it, if the eye were not in some measure the sun, it could not know the sun.

In addition to the physical body, other manifestations of the physical world are being transcribed into music. Computer scientist Robert C. Morrison of East Carolina University in North Carolina has developed computer programs that will translate patterns of numerical data into musical tones. He points out that the ear is a much more sensitive instrument than the eye for recognizing patterns. Thus through the medium of music a person could distinguish recurrent themes in chemical analyses, economic indicators, and other patterns of data too complex to allow ready analysis either visually or mathematically. In quality control systems, an investigator could listen for disharmonies in the music instead of looking for mathematical irregularities.[17]

The physical world also can be experienced by bringing the sense of touch into play. Scientists David W. Abraham, Ralph L. Hollis, and Septimiu E. Salcudean at the IBM Thomas J. Watson Research

Center in Yorktown Heights, New York, have developed a "magic wrist" that converts complex images from a scanning electron microscope, an instrument that can display the surface atoms of a material, into three-dimensional movements. This permits the person wearing the wrist device actually to feel the atomic surface structures of metals and alloys. The IBM group plans also to attach their magic wrist to an atomic-force microscope, which measures the attractive forces binding metals together, to enable people to experience firsthand the affinities between the constituent chemicals.[18] This will allow the investigator to feel what is going on at the atomic level—literally to "have a feeling" for the substance with which he or she is working.

Similar attempts have been made in medicine and surgery. One eye surgeon is seeking to apply the magic wrist in doing retinal surgery. Presumably anything that would magnify one's sense of touch would create an advantage in performing delicate surgical procedures, which now are done by relying primarily on vision. This would be like having one's fingertips in the cutting edge of the scalpel.[19]

One can imagine a multisensory device that not only would transcribe the body's DNA into music as Ohno has done, but translate it into kinesthetic stimuli as well—a kind of "magic ear" and "magic wrist" combined. This would allow us to hear *and* feel what is going on inside our DNA and other body parts, allowing grander visions of the body than anything contained in the machine view.

One can also imagine diagnostic devices that make use of these capabilities. Today the various X-ray and scanning devices give the physician primarily visual images of the function of certain organs—thyroid, lung, liver, kidney, and others. Based on the appearance of those images, the physician judges whether or not the organ "looks" normal. But rather than diagnosticians saying only that there appears to be a spot on the lung or a mass in the liver, the new devices might enable them to detect bodily disharmonies using nonvisual senses—to say, for example, that the lung tissue sounds out of key, that there are sour notes coming from the thyroid, or that the kidney is off beat—or, while wearing the magic wrist, to say that these organs literally do not feel right.

Today the practice of medicine is regarded largely as an intellectual affair. These diagnostic methods would go far beyond the intellect, however, and engage the senses and sensitivities of the physician in a much broader way. Although they would make the practice of medicine more demanding, they almost certainly would bring new meaning and greater fulfillment to being a doctor because they would call forth more of his or her innate human potential. And these breakthroughs just might make the practice of medicine easier. Just as the introduction of the stethoscope expanded what physicians could hear, these new tools would expand the reach of the senses and thus provide the physician with more information on which to base his or her judgments.

Physiologist Robert S. Root-Bernstein of Michigan State University has written of the need for a *sensual science*. Tools such as those above could revolutionize the way physicians and young scientists in general perceive the physical world. They would speed discovery, he suggests, because they would enhance the creative process by allowing a firsthand, immediate knowledge of the natural world. Root-Bernstein points out that many of the greatest scientists had the ability to relate sensually to their object of investigation. A typical recent example is Nobel Prize–winning geneticist Barbara McClintock, who attributed her astonishing insights to a highly developed "feeling for the organism." Another Nobelist, the great neuroanatomist and histologist Santiago Ramón y Cajal, also possessed this ability. Sir Charles Sherrington, the legendary English neurologist who studied with Ramón y Cajal, reported: "He treated the microscopic scene as though it were alive and were inhabited by beings which felt and did and hoped and tried even as we do. . . . He would envisage the sperm cells as activated by a sort of passionate urge in their rivalry for penetration into the ovum-cell."[20]

Sherrington, one of the greatest neurologists in the history of medicine, was himself able to see the body in highly novel ways. He coined one of the most endearing terms to describe the human brain—the "enchanted loom"—which, in the context of the body as music, translates easily into a musical instrument: a magic harp, lyre, piano.

In his admirable book *Nada Brahma: The World Is Sound,* musicologist and writer Joachim-Ernst Berendt observes that in Latin the term meaning "to sound through something" is *personare*. "Thus," he states,

> at the basis of the concept of the *person* . . . stands a concept of sound: "through the tone." If nothing sounds through from the bottom of the being, a human being is human biologically, at best, but is not a *per-son,* because he does not live through the *son* (the tone, the sound). He does not live the sound which is the world.[21]

The trick is to hear the music that is the body. If we can do so, the meaning of the body can be transformed. It becomes not a blind, silent, doomed machine but a glorious composition, a part of God's oeuvre: the Great Tone.

PART THREE

HEALING BREAK-THROUGHS

Meaning makes a great many things endurable— perhaps everything. [Through] the creation of meaning . . . a new cosmos arises.

—C. G. JUNG[1]

The Case of the Fishskin Boy:
Genes and Memes

In the early 1950s a sixteen-year-old English boy with a severe case of "warts" visited a surgeon, seeking their removal. The warts, however, were too extensive for surgery to be of help, and the surgeon declined to treat him. Instead he suggested hypnosis, because he knew that hypnosis can be very effective in getting rid of warts, although nobody knows how. Thus, after taking a biopsy of the affected skin, the surgeon referred the boy to an anesthesiologist, Dr. A. A. Mason, who used hypnosis in his practice.

The boy was severely afflicted with thickened, scaly, deformed, and fissured skin covering almost all his body. Infection was so extensive and foul smelling he could not attend school. Dr. Mason found the boy to be an excellent hypnotic candidate and agreed to treat him with hypnosis. After he was hypnotized, Mason suggested to him that the thickened, disfigured, infected skin disappear, one extremity at a time, and be replaced by healthy, pink, normal skin.

Then, at a case conference at his hospital the next day, the situation took an unexpected turn. Mason was surprised to learn from the pathologists who had examined the biopsy that the diagnosis had been wrong: this was not warts but a severe case of congenital ichthyosis, or "fishskin" disease.

What was Mason to do? There is no known physical treatment for

this genetic disease, let alone therapy based on "powers of the mind."
But what harm could be done? Mason decided to continue the hypnosis.

Mason's hypnotic suggestions brought results. He extended this
treatment from the extremities to the entire body. Soon, for the first time
in his life, the boy had healthy-appearing skin.

Dr. Henry L. Bennett, of the University of California School of
Medicine at Davis, describes the boy's subsequent course: "At follow-ups
of one month and four years, the treatments resulted in a 60 to 70
percent permanent improvement of the skin. Photographs throughout the
treatments documented the change, and dermatologic and pathological
analysis confirmed that the disorder was a congenital ichthyosis. Mason
published his report in the *British Medical Journal*. By noon of publication
day, the journal had to open a special switchboard to receive calls from
as far away as India."[1]

Lewis Thomas, chancellor of Sloan-Kettering Cancer Center in New
York, has been called "the most listened-to physician in America."
For him, the fact that warts (the disease Mason originally thought he
was treating), which are caused by a virus, can disappear under the
mind's influence is astonishing and highly important. It even de-
serves, he suggests, a "National Institute of Warts" to investigate it.
Thomas believes that the warts respond because of an inner power in
all of us—"a kind of superintelligence" or an inner "controller." The
ability to self-heal is activated when we make contact with these
forces.[2]

A key to this boy's breakthrough was the fact that he was highly
hypnotizable. Most authorities on hypnosis view this as a key to good
results. In one study, a practitioner treated 121 asthma patients with
hypnosis over a ten-year span. Those who were cured (defined as
regaining normal breathing capacity) were the ones who were highly
hypnotizable. Those not helped were not hypnotizable. In another
study involving 100 patients with migraine treated with hypnosis, the
23 who became symptom free were all capable of medium or deep
levels of hypnosis.[3]

The ability to be deeply hypnotized seems to be fairly stable from
childhood onward. Children who were highly active in building
fantasies and using their imaginations, and who found these experi-

ences satisfying and pleasurable, are likely to be good hypnotic candidates. Also adding to this ability are adventuresomeness and activities like reading, listening to music, and performing. These activities all suggest a fundamental ability to ignore distractions, "dissociate," and become totally immersed in the experience at hand.[4]

Thomas's view that the mind could play a powerful role in combating an infectious disease is generally not shared by physicians. Even more heretical is the possibility that the mind could intervene in genetic diseases. Physicians believe that, perhaps, thoughts and emotions might make a difference in some illnesses, but they do not affect those that are genetic in origin. Doctors generally believe that the genes are simply off-limits, beyond the reach of the mind. They are considered the absolute, omnipotent dictators of the physical body. This point of view was vividly described in 1976 by the Oxford biologist Richard Dawkins in his book *The Selfish Gene*. Dawkins proposed that we are all—no exceptions—slaves.[5] "Humans are nothing but temporary survival machines, robot vehicles blindly programmed for someone else's benefit," he said. The real rulers of human beings are the tiny bits of DNA that make up our genes. So "ruthless" and "selfish" are our genes that Dawkins compared them to a Chicago gangster mob. Their sole aim is their own perpetuation, and they will stop at nothing to attain it.

On the surface this message seems extremely depressing and disempowering. It suggests that all our ideas about freedom of choice, the higher emotions such as love, and virtues such as altruism and sacrifice are hallucinations created by the genes themselves. We are merely machines on automatic pilot; the control system is not our minds but our DNA. Our genes have ironically permitted us to *believe* we are free, but this is only the final link in our chain of total enslavement.

But unlike a genetic determinist, Dawkins ends his book with this stunning sentence: "We, alone on earth, can rebel against the tyranny of the selfish replicators." We can break the domination of the genes and escape our enslavement. How? In addition to genes, Dawkins posits another unit of evolution, the *meme*. Memes are bits of consciousness. Unlike genes, which are "blind" and unconscious, memes have awareness and foresight. They are ideas, thoughts, imaginings, beliefs. Memes are *meanings*. And, like genes, they are capable of perpetuating themselves, flowing down through time, generation after generation.

Dawkins believes that, within limits, we can choose between the influence of genes or memes and that this is what distinguishes humans from lower animals.[6] A commonplace example is the decision to use contraception. Anytime anyone decides to thwart conception, the invisible replicators are stopped dead in their tracks because their "blind," "ruthless," "selfish" program for survival and perpetuation is derailed. Momentarily, at any rate, we have escaped their tyranny and are not their slaves. And what has allowed our temporary freedom? It is *meaning*—what "pregnancy," "family size," and "parenthood" *mean* to us, how we *interpret* them, the *significance* they hold for us. We may translate these meanings into other terms, calling them "beliefs" or "opinions," but in the end it is what these concepts *mean* to us that counts.

The case of the sixteen-year-old boy whose genetic disease responded to hypnosis is an example of the power of "bits of consciousness," in the form of meanings, to break the domination of the genes. If the boy had allowed "gene" to mean something totally dominant against which he was helpless, it would likely have been impossible for him to enter the deep level of hypnosis; he could not genuinely have believed, imaged, or fantasized that normal skin would replace the thickened, genetically blighted skin. But a new meme, a new "bit of consciousness"—a new meaning—allowed the healing images to flourish.

Skeptics argue that thoughts cannot change genes, but that is not the point. *People suffering from genetic diseases need not change the genes themselves, only their manifestations.* Presumably no one would argue that the "fishskin boy" actually changed his genes through thought. But he did change their *expression*, which seems the most important point.

It is important that persons with certain genetically related medical problems be presented this positive approach; otherwise they may be denied access to potentially helpful methods of therapy.

Max was a thirty-five-year-old computer engineer. I first met him when he was in the hospital emergency room following a heart attack. He suffered from familial hypercholesterolemia, a genetic disorder associated with high blood cholesterol and early death from heart disease. Because every male in his family had died in his thirties from heart attack, Max was highly motivated to make changes in his health patterns. By the time I met him he had become a vegetarian, adopted a rigorous program of physical activity, lowered his body weight to an ideal level, and adhered religiously to a program of cholesterol-lowering medications.

Although his recovery was uneventful, he became extremely depressed following discharge from the hospital. He had done everything his previous physicians had advised and was rewarded with a myocardial infarction. Now he saw his fate sealed by his genes, just like all the males in his family before him.

"Let's start over," I suggested to him, "and look at things afresh." We reviewed his records and saw that the things he had done—diet, exercise, weight loss, and medications—had resulted in some lowering of his cholesterol level. "Look," I pointed out, "your body is very sensitive to what *you* do. Although still high, your cholesterol *has* come down; it *does* get the message. And there are more messages you can give it."

"Like what?" he asked skeptically.

I reviewed with him the evidence that, in men with genetically based high cholesterol levels, the levels frequently fell by about one-third when a program of quiet relaxation was adopted.[7] This program involved no esoteric techniques, only sitting serenely for twice a day, twenty minutes each time, allowing any thought that might enter the mind to pass.

Max wasn't convinced. "If the genes don't respond to the *physical* things I've done, what can 'doing nothing' possibly do?" Still, he agreed to try, and I referred him to the biofeedback laboratory to learn the basic skills of quiet relaxation.

His response was typical of persons studied scientifically who pursued this technique: his cholesterol level fell approximately one-third, to a below-average level. Max reappraised his previous idea that thoughts and "doing nothing" could not influence the way his genes were directing his body. He continues to employ all the physically based methods in addition to quiet relaxation and clearing the mind. Ten years following his heart attack he has had no further problems, his cholesterol level remains below normal, and he has set the record for longevity for males in his family.

There is evidence in scientific studies in bacteria that *the genes of an individual cell can profit by experience and that the meaning or significance of an event actually can change them.* Harvard's John Cairns and his co-workers placed bacteria that were incapable of utilizing the sugar lactose in a solution in which there was no other available nutrient. In order to consume the lactose and avoid starving, they had to mutate at a higher-than-normal rate. This they did, and they passed the ability to consume lactose on to future generations.[8] Researcher Barry Hall at the University of Connecticut subjected bacteria to an even more difficult task. In order to metabolize the sugar that was their only nutrient, they had to perform two mutations, one of which was an excision of existing genetic instructions. The odds against the two mutations occurring randomly during the same time period are more than one in a trillion. As in Cairns' experiment, the bacteria performed the mutations and passed on the newly acquired ability to subsequent generations of organisms.[9]

These findings make many geneticists and molecular biologists uncomfortable. They raise the possibility of Lamarckism, the long-discarded idea that acquired characteristics can alter the genetic structure and be forwarded via DNA to future generations. They suggest also that our basic units of inheritance, our DNA, may be sensitive to the *meaning* of a situation—its significance and importance for the organism. If so, we may be wrong in believing that only higher organisms such as ourselves respond to meaning and that meaning is perceived only through complex structures such as human brains. If *bacteria* can catch the meaning or significance of a situation and adapt to it by changing their DNA, this ability may be spread throughout the biological world from the simplest organisms to the most complex. In which case we underestimate ourselves if we assume always that our genes have the last word.

To summarize the lessons we can learn from these extraordinary findings and the case of the fishskin boy:

- Genes are not destiny. They do not have the final word in how the body behaves. The manifestations of consciousness—emotions, thoughts, feeling states, perceived meanings—are also involved.

- We should be careful about the meanings we allow "gene" and "genetic" to hold for us, for these meanings determine what we deem to be possible, and can either enhance or interfere with healing.
- Certain states of consciousness such as deep hypnosis, in which our everyday awareness leaves the stage, can activate our inner "superintelligence" and allow dramatic self-healing to occur.

One of the methods of activating this superintelligence, this innate capacity for healing, is the ancient practice of psychic healing, which we will now examine.

The Power of Belief:
Psychic Healing and the Harvard Health Service

The mind, in addition to medicine, has powers to
turn the immune system around. . . .

—JONAS SALK[1]

Harvard psychologist David McClelland advised thirteen Harvard undergraduates with common colds to go to a psychic healer in the Boston area
within twenty-four hours after the onset of symptoms. The psychic healer
kept the "therapy" simple, saying only "You're healed" to each student.

To assess the effect of this "treatment," McClelland designed a list
of thirty-two symptoms which indicated the severity of the illness before
and after the treatment. He also measured the levels of an antibody,
immunoglobulin A (IgA), in the subjects' saliva. (IgA helps combat upper
respiratory illnesses such as colds.) The results: following the healing
ritual, nine of the thirteen students who felt their colds get better also
demonstrated higher levels of IgA. Therefore, not only did they get
better symptomatically, but their subjective improvement correlated with
measurable physical changes.

When word got around about McClelland's unorthodox experiment,
the physicians at the Harvard University Health Service became irritated.
They told McClelland that the results really had nothing to do with the

psychic healer, and that he would get the same results if he would send the students to the health service and allow the M.D.'s to tell them they would get better. McClelland took up the challenge and repeated the experiment, this time letting the health service doctors tell the sick student that he or she would improve. But no student saw any improvement, and neither did the IgA antibody levels change.[2]

As McClelland showed, a belief is not simply "mental," not some ethereal entity floating around the head, hovering mistily somewhere above the clavicles. Beliefs permeate and actually change the body. They bring about concrete changes that can easily be measured.

The nature of the belief is sometimes unimportant. Often the body simply doesn't care if the therapy is legitimate and accepted or outrageous and unorthodox, as the following two cases show.

Dr. Myrin Borysenko was for many years a prominent researcher in immunology at Tufts University School of Medicine. His area of expertise was the interaction of the psyche and the brain with the neurological and immune systems. He knew of McClelland's experiment in psychic healing with the Harvard students, and on one occasion had discussed his findings with him. "How does the healer do it?" he asked. McClelland simply replied, "Oh, he just messes with your mind."

One morning, while at work in his laboratory, Myrin began to come down with symptoms of flu—fever, aches, cough, and congestion. He had colds and the flu often, and invariably they kept him off work for a week. By noon he felt miserable and could not function well. He decided to leave work and go home to bed.

On his way home he suddenly thought of McClelland's experiment. Why not give the psychic healer a try? After all, he reasoned, there's no good alternative treatment, and no one will ever know.

Myrin found the healer's address in a dilapidated part of the city. As he climbed the rickety stairs he began to have second thoughts. What if my colleagues could see me now? he said to himself. The door to the healer's apartment was open as if Myrin were expected. He entered to find an enormously fat, unkempt man sprawled on a sofa watching a soap opera on TV and drinking wine from a gallon jug.

Summoning his courage, Myrin said, "I hear you can cure people. Can you cure my flu?"

Without taking his eyes off the TV, the healer said, "No problem." He reached for a small bottle of purple liquid on the floor. "Go into the bathroom, fill the tub half full of water, pour this stuff in, and sit in it for thirty minutes. Then you will be cured."

Myrin did as he was told. As he sat in the tub, up to his waist in the densely purple water, he was struck by the sheer absurdity of what he was doing. There is something preposterous about an academic immunologist seeking a cure for the flu from a wine-guzzling psychic healer, he thought. He felt so utterly silly that he started to laugh uncontrollably. He could not stop. He was still laughing when he realized his half-hour was over.

Myrin dressed and walked to the living room to find the healer still engrossed in the soap opera. Again without looking at him he simply said, "Now you are healed." Then he pointed to the door, indicating that Myrin was free to go.

Driving home, Myrin slowly realized that things were different. He sensed no fever and his headache had disappeared. Gone also were the cough, congestion, and body aches. He felt good—so good, in fact, that he decided to return to work.

Myrin worked late. As he was reciting his tale that night to his wife while undressing for bed, she suddenly burst into laughter. Looking into the mirror he knew why. He was purple from the waist down.[3]

A physician reported his experience with three patients—one with inoperable cancer of the uterus, another with chronic gallbladder disease, and a third with severe pancreatitis. On his own, he contacted a local faith healer who could reputedly send strong healing energy to persons at a distance. The healer agreed to intercede for the patients, completely unknown to them. However, after twelve sessions they were no better, and the healer went out of town and stopped the procedure. Only then did the physician approach his patients and tell them of this healer who could help them. He said that on a certain day they would receive powerful healing forces from him. The doctor continued to "talk up" the treatment. All three patients began improving almost immediately. The patient with cancer experienced an impressive remission. She was able to resume her activities as a housewife and mother. Although she died three months later, she was happier, more active, and free of pain. The gallbladder patient was sent home from the hospital free of pain and remained symptom free for a year. The woman with pancreatitis got out of bed, gained thirty pounds, and recovered completely.[4]

Psychologist and author Lawrence LeShan studied psychic healing for many years. He interviewed and observed some of the most skillful healers on several continents. He concluded from his research that, although patients were occasionally healed while interacting with psychic healers, "there [is] no such thing as psychic healing. There [is] only self-healing, [which can] sometimes . . . be potentiated by the action of the healer." When we are sick, "we are in a weakened condition, unable to use our self-healing abilities to their fullest. The specialized interaction of psychic healing changes this. . . . If conditions are right (and we know very little about what that means), the healee joins in, nourishes a part of himself that is undernourished, and is, for a time, more complete and better able to use his own self-healing abilities."[5] LeShan seems to be referring to these same self-healing abilities that Lewis Thomas called the "superintelligence" and "inner controller" in all of us.

Psychic healing takes many forms. While some healers go to great lengths and use bizarre methods to "mess up the mind," as the healer studied by McClelland above, this is usually *not* the form psychic healing takes. Following LeShan, we can say that psychic healing occurs anytime someone's self-healing capacity is potentiated by another. It is likely that most of us function as psychic healers from time to time without realizing it. And most of us *receive* psychic healing periodically, also without knowing it. This is illustrated in the following case, reported by University of Michigan nurse-theorists and educators Helen C. Erickson, Evelyn M. Tomlin, and Mary Ann P. Swain. In it, a concerned husband unknowingly acts as a psychic healer for his unconscious wife. This case is instructive for another reason: it shows that psychic healing can bypass the conscious mind of the patient. For this reason, psychic healing cannot be explained away as mere power of suggestion.

A thirty-four-year-old mother of three children had severe headaches. She was found to have a glioma, a malignant brain tumor, and was taken to surgery where the tumor was found to be inoperable. While she lay in coma in the postoperative period, the discouraged surgeon told her husband, "There is nothing more we can do." The husband recalled the spectacular recovery of actress Patricia Neal from a stroke, and stubbornly refused to go along with the surgeon's proclamation. "Oh, yes, there is! you *will* do surgery and you *will* do chemotherapy!" he said. The husband resolutely stationed himself at his unconscious wife's bedside and maintained a constant vigil. He talked to her, stroked her hand, kept her informed about what was happening with their children, and shared his plans for life ahead. "I know you can't respond," he told her. "It probably makes you feel very bad. But you will be better, and you will be part of our family again." The nurses on the unit were sympathetic, but the woman's situation was so dismal they did not share the husband's hopes. "Poor fellow," they said. "He's taking this so hard. He probably needs his denial for a time." Five days after surgery the woman began to stir. Slowly but surely she began to recover, astonishing everyone but her husband. Finally she went home, returning at three-month intervals. A full two years later, at last report, she was doing very well and had just been told by her physician that her most recent brain scan was normal.[6]

It is becoming clear that almost anyone can liberate and potentiate the "superintelligence" or inner healing capacity of someone in need. This means that we all may be psychic healers—including, as the following research suggests, orthodox physicians who might even deny that psychic healing exists.

At a rehabilitation hospital in Chicago, a group of researchers tested the effects of a spoken message on patients undergoing back surgery. The patients were unconscious, under total anesthesia, and presumably had no awareness that a message was being spoken.

The commonest complication following surgery of this type is the inability to urinate voluntarily. This is treated by the temporary insertion of a urinary catheter. To avoid this, the researchers tried another solution. Toward the end of surgery, while the patient was still anesthetized, the surgeon spoke to the patient by name and said:

The operation has gone well and we will soon be finishing. You will be flat on your back for the next couple of days. When you are waiting it would be a good idea if you relax the muscles in the pelvic area. This will help you to urinate, so you won't need a catheter.

The results were impressive. Not a single patient given this suggestion required a catheter after surgery. More than half those in a control group, not given the suggestion, needed catheterization.[7]

Another group of medical researchers made the point more dramatically that suggestions given under anesthesia can later be recalled and acted upon. During an operation a tape was played through earphones worn by the anesthetized patients, suggesting that when a researcher came to interview them afterward, "it is very important that you pull on your ear so I can know you have heard this." During the interviews, more than 80 percent of the patients who heard that suggestion pulled at their ears; most of them did so six times or more.[8]

Again, these events show that healing can be brought about by a variety of people, even those who might never call themselves "psychic" healers, and that the healing can be mediated by the unconscious, unaware part of the mind.

Psychic healing does not always originate outside ourselves. It can come from within. By our own beliefs we can potentiate our healing systems and set our innate superintelligence in action.

One of the most dramatic examples of this process is the well-known placebo response. A placebo is a bogus pill, with no known biological effect. Yet the power of placebos is legendary. They are as effective as morphine in relieving severe pain in a significant percentage of the population.

One of my earliest exposures to the power of placebos came when working in a hospital pharmacy during college. The chief pharmacist seemed continually to be compounding a medication called Lipragus. Lipragus was the most popular medication in the hospital. It was being ordered for patients in the coronary care unit, surgery wards, obstetric floors, and medical units. I thought it strange that I had never heard of this medication. Neither could I imagine how a single drug could have such vast applicability. I looked up Lipragus in the pharmacology reference books and could not find it. I was surprised also to find it missing in the *Physician's Desk Reference,* which lists all the prescription drugs available in the United States. Confused, I sought out the chief pharmacist and asked him to tell me about Lipragus. "Quite simple," he said. "It's 'sugar pill' spelled backward. For years it has been the hottest drug in the hospital!"

Sir William Osler, who is frequently described as the father of scientific medicine in the United States, once said, "The desire to take medicine is perhaps the greatest feature which distinguishes man from animals."[9] In addition to wanting to *take* medicine, of course we want it to *work.* This is what makes the placebo response so potent.

The importance of one's belief system on the action of drugs became widely appreciated in America in the counterculture of the sixties, when psychedelic drugs became popular. It was soon recognized that whether the drug effect was pleasant or unpleasant was not due entirely to the drug itself. Something besides the chemical was involved, something that could change a good trip into a bad one, and vice versa. In perfect accord with what the street-smart enthusiasts of psychedelics had reported, professional psychologists later distinguished between the "set" and "setting." The set was the drug itself—its chemical makeup and dosage—and the setting was the "soft" factors such as the actual location of the experience, the people involved, and the overall meaning and significance of the experience for the person.

To many, "drug experience" conjures images of crazed addicts, "crack" houses, murder, and mayhem. But this concept is too narrow: we all "do" drugs in one form or another—alcohol, aspirin, vitamins; the list is endless. Because the habit of ingesting foreign substances is ubiquitous, "set" and "setting" are issues for everyone.

A well-documented example of how these factors operate comes from mushroom picking, a hobby enjoyed by millions of persons in this country and around the world. Writer Wade Davis describes what can happen:

> In the northwest rain forest of Oregon there are a number of hallucinogenic mushrooms. Those who go out into the forest deliberately *intending* to ingest these mushrooms generally experience a pleasant intoxication. Those who *inadvertently* consume them while foraging for edible

mushrooms invariably end up in the nearest hospital. The mushroom itself has not changed [emphasis added].[10]

Here, as in the following example, what comes to the fore as the key factor is—the *meaning* of the experience for the person his belief system.

Michael Harner, the noted anthropologist, is renowned for his books and workshops about shamanism. In the opening session of one of the workshops, he discussed the role of hallucinogenic plants in producing the shaman's trance state and his ecstatic "journey to other worlds," whereby he gains knowledge that is useful in healing sick persons in his community. Since this was an experiential workshop, Harner told the twenty students that he wanted them to have a firsthand experience of the shaman's altered states of consciousness, at which point he produced a wrinkled paper sack from which he removed a desiccated, fibrous root. He announced that ingesting the substance was purely optional: no one was required to do it if they had strong feelings against it. He then twisted off a small amount of the root, ate it, and passed the root to his left, adding that one should be careful not to take too much. Soon the root had made the rounds, with everyone taking a portion. Harner announced that it would take about an hour for the full effect to occur. In the meantime the students were to go outdoors and experience nature with the maximal attention possible, fully noticing the shapes of leaves, the touch of flower petals, the reflections in dew.

At the end of the hour the twenty students and Harner reassembled indoors. The altered state of consciousness was much in evidence. Some persons were ecstatic, some were clearly intoxicated, some were having visions. Harner asked each person to relate what the experience was like. In turn, each gave his or her description of how the world had changed. Without exception, everyone reported that colors were brighter, the touch of leaves on the skin was electric, smells were intensely stimulating, the presence of others was magical, and a sense of joy pervaded everything. For everyone, the whole world was excruciatingly wonderful!

By this time, the curiosity of the group about the identity of the mind-expanding vegetable matter was overwhelming. But Harner seemed hesitant to reveal its identity. Finally, with much prodding, he agreed. "The substance you ate," he said slowly, "was ginger root."

The room was stunned and silent. Everyone realized they'd been tricked. Ingesting a common spice found in millions of kitchens across America had catapulted them into the most ecstatic trance they'd ever experienced. Then Harner, after allowing the lesson to sink in, began his deep, booming laugh. The atmosphere lightened and the group began to laugh with him.

Harner demonstrated one of the most fundamental facts of shamanic reality: our experience of the world heavily depends on our attitudes *about* it—again, our belief system in action.

Some people think that the belief system affects only placebos or weak medications but that the effects of belief can be overridden by extremely potent drugs. Evidence suggests this is not true, and that the emotions and attitudes surrounding the ingestion of very powerful drugs can create life-or-death effects.

At Ontario's McMaster University, researcher Shepard Siegel and his colleagues performed a series of experiments in which two groups of rats, each in a distinct environment, were injected with small but increasing doses of heroin. They developed a tolerance for the drug and became addicted to it. Then the rats in one group were taken from their cage and put in an unfamiliar setting, while the other group was kept in their accustomed environment. Both groups were then given another injection of heroin at a dosage they had previously tolerated quite well. Although the dose remained the same, many of those rats who were moved to the new surroundings died from it, while those who remained in their original cage tolerated it as usual.[11]

Siegel points out that animals become adapted to the stimuli of the environment (sights, sounds, smells, etc.) and these stimuli become part of the overall effects of the drug. As a general rule, new environmental stimuli appear to increase the sensitivity to the drug, familiar surroundings to diminish it.

What are the implications for humans? Siegel believes drugs may have a more pronounced effect in us if taken in an unfamiliar context. He interviewed addicts in a methadone clinic in New York and found considerable evidence to support this idea. The stories he uncovered were consistent with the anecdotal observations everyone is familiar with: overdose victims frequently are found in places unfamiliar to them—hotel rooms, back streets, public rest rooms, alleys, and so on.

No one has yet compared the effects of prescription drugs taken in unfamiliar surroundings such as hospitals or while on vacation to their effects when taken in the privacy and familiarity of one's own home. Siegel's studies, however, suggest that we might see significant differences. It might make a difference, for example, if chemotherapy drugs are given in a reassuring, homey environment rather than in a sterile, stainless-steel-and-glass atmosphere that reeks of antiseptic. This suggests an entirely new way of thinking about the side effects of a drug. Not only should we be concerned about the dosage given, or whether or not a true sensitivity or allergy to the chemical exists, but in addition we should be attentive to the overall meaning and significance of the experience for the person who is ingesting it.

HEART DISEASE: CREATING NEW MEANINGS

Heart disease is the number one killer in the United States. It causes more deaths than all other diseases combined. It is perhaps in heart disease that the power of belief and meaning—of what we feel and think about the disease—is most vivid.

The meanings and beliefs of persons who have heart disease are not set in stone. They are malleable, and new ones can be created that are health giving and lifesaving. With changes in meaning can come, literally, a change of heart.

Dr. Meyer Friedman and his colleagues at Mount Zion Hospital Medical Center of the University of California, San Francisco and Stanford University studied 1,035 consecutive patients who survived their heart attacks to determine if they could alter their "Type A" behavior, and whether or not this alteration would make a difference in subsequent survival. They found that more than ninety-eight percent of all the

patients exhibited Type A behavior, the emotional syndrome characterized by a continuously harassing sense of time urgency and easily
aroused hostility and cynicism. For true Type A's there is never enough
time to get things done, and they direct anger outward—toward traffic
lights that turn red, waiters who don't come on time, spouses and
children who aren't perfect, and on and on.[12]

About 300 of Friedman's subjects received the typical advice given
to patients who have had a heart attack—information on diet and body
weight, the importance of exercise, etc. Another 600 patients also
received this advice, but in addition were shown—through psychological
counseling, biofeedback teaching, and individual and group education—how to change their Type A behavior. The remaining patients,
about 150, received no counseling but were examined and interviewed
annually by their physicians.

The study continued for five years. During this time some of the
subjects had recurrent heart attacks, some of which were fatal. Others
died suddenly, "dropping dead" from cardiac arrest presumably due to
their heart disease. It was found that the circumstances most often
preceding these events were emotional crises, excessive physical activity,
consumption of a large fatty meal, or some combination of these
circumstances.

When the statistics were examined at the end of one year, the rates
of nonfatal heart attacks were lowest in the group given in-depth
instruction on modifying their Type A behavior. In contrast, the group
receiving the typical advice about diet, weight, and exercise had three
times, and the control group four times, as many nonfatal heart attacks.
In addition, the in-depth group had less than half the number of fatal
heart attacks as the control group.

What happened to the patients who underwent the in-depth training?
Their program was essentially a kind of "meaning therapy" because
it helped them gain new interpretations of everyday life events: If the
morning paper is tossed in the mud, if I'm late for an appointment, or
if my teenager doesn't make straight As, it is hardly the end of the
world. Even if I'm passed over for a promotion, someone crashes
into my car, or my house burns down, I shall survive. With the
creation of new meanings, the body responds in healthier ways. The
"adrenaline rush" that is felt in a crisis is blunted, along with the rise
in heart rate and blood pressure. The diffuse anxiety and hostility

Type As feel throughout the day abates, and the body's "emergency" apparatus, the sympathetic nervous system, is quieted. One of the primary benefactors of these changes is the heart.

This important study shows that

- meanings can be changed,
- the significance that life events hold for us is *not* absolute, and
- as the meanings change to a more positive outlook, the rate of recurrent heart attack declines.[13]

Successful results from modifying behaviors in heart patients were also found by cardiologist Dean Ornish. Ornish taught stress management techniques to twenty-three patients who had heart disease, and compared them over a twenty-four-day period to an equal number of similar patients who were not taught these methods. (All forty-six patients were given a diet very low in fat.) The stress management techniques consisted of stretching and relaxation exercises; meditation (sitting quietly, breathing slowly and deeply, and returning to a focus on breathing when the mind wandered); and visualization in which the subject imagined, while meditating, that the cholesterol deposits were being removed from his or her arteries.

The results of the twenty-four-day study were significant. In the stress management group there was a 44 percent mean increase in the duration of exercise, a 55 percent increase in total work performed, and improved function of the left ventricle of the heart when assessed by objective methods that measure the motion of the ventricular wall of the heart. In addition the researchers noted a 20 percent fall in cholesterol levels and a 90 percent reduction in the frequency of attacks of angina, the pain associated with coronary artery disease.[14]

What happened emotionally to patients who engaged in meditation and visualization? As in the above study by Friedman, these methods can be viewed as *meaning therapies*. As many persons who have successfully participated in any of these methods know, one's way of being in the world shifts. Events that previously were stressful cease to feel burdensome because they are no longer individualized by a defensive ego that is constantly seeking to ensure its own security.

For example, life no longer seems unfair just because the rent is increased, the tax rate rises, or ten traffic lights in a row turn red. Tolerance for complexity increases as events seem to fit together in harmonious patterns that previously were invisible. The result is an increased resiliency of the psyche and an emotional durability that allows one to roll with the punches. Again, the result for the heart patient is improved cardiac function and fewer heart attacks.

Many persons feel that these benefits are too good to be true. They believe that to change deeply ingrained meanings, years of work in therapy must be required. That frequently has been the message from modern psychiatry: deep, "real" change can come about only with prolonged effort. To be sure, changing many aspects of the psyche is time consuming and laborious. But this is by no means true of all its aspects. In Ornish's study, striking benefits to both mind and body were obvious in only twenty-four days!

All the case studies in this chapter have dealt with the operation of the belief system within a single person—the effects on *my* body and *my* health of *my* beliefs. This may seem to suggest that the power of belief operates only when we are concerned about our own welfare. But as we will now see, the healing power of the belief system can, paradoxically, be set in motion when we are concerned not about ourselves but others.

The Helper's High:
Healing the Self
by Helping Others

When the experiences of over 1,700 women who were involved regularly in helping others were analyzed at the Institute for the Advancement of Health (I.A.H.) in New York City, they revealed relief of actual physical ailments in the wake of the helping. Disorders such as headaches, loss of voice, pain due to lupus and multiple sclerosis, and depression improved.[1]

Helping others is a door through which one can walk at any time "to forget oneself," as Harvard cardiologist Herbert Benson puts it. This forgetting of the self is frequently associated with pleasant bodily sensations. These sensations are so distinctive they have been given a name: the "helper's high."

In two surveys 68 and 88 percent of persons [doing volunteer work] reported an identifiable physical sensation during the actual helping. One woman described it as "a gentle tightness in my chest and neck, like an increased blood flow." Another compared it to her "sense of fitness and well-being" she feels while swimming. And a nursing home volunteer likened it to the good, tired feeling she has after a game of tennis. Many women described a greater calmness and an enhanced sense of self-worth following the helping.[2]

Researchers have noted the similarities between the helper's high and the high frequently described by long-distance runners. "Runner's high" has been linked to an increase in the body's levels of endorphins, our natural opiates. The same explanation may lie behind the helper's high. As psychologist Jaak Panksepp of Bowling Green State University states, based on his and other experiments, "It is just about proven that it is our own natural opiates, the endorphins, that produce the good feelings that arise during social contact with others."[3]

But unlike the runner's high, the helper's high can be turned on at will. In his survey of women who helped others, I.A.H.'s Allan Luks discovered that 82 percent said their helper's high would recur, though with less intensity, when they simply remembered helping.

Some people learn to use the helper's high therapeutically.

One woman, for example, discovered that her volunteer work at a nursing home could be used to keep her blood pressure under control. Thirteen percent of all persons in the I.A.H. survey noted a decrease in aches and pains as a result of helping. Almost 90 percent felt that their health was better than, or as good as, others their age.

Forgetting oneself through altruistic behavior seems to require actual human contact. An impersonal act, like writing a check to a charitable organization, does not seem to initiate the process. As a volunteer who made recordings for the blind said, "They're important. But I only feel that good high when I'm with others, like assisting the free-lunch program." It also seems necessary that the altruism be given freely and not out of a sense of obligation. People who have long-term caring duties for the elderly and who cannot escape them have more, not less, health problems, and they rarely report the helper's high. And the helping must fit into an overall, harmonious pattern. As one student put it, when her volunteer activities interfere with her studies, they cease to be rewarding.[4]

Maggie was twenty years old, a third-year student in a local university, and a "candystriper"—a hospital volunteer, so called because of the red-striped uniform worn by all the volunteer staff. When I initially met her in the hospital emergency room—her first night as an E.R. volunteer—she was not tolerating her experience well.

Four automobile accident victims had arrived simultaneously, two of whom were mangled beyond recognition and dead on arrival. The remaining two were in critical condition. They were semiconscious, had multiple fractures, were covered with blood, and had grotesque, disfiguring facial lacerations. The scene was chaotic. All hands were needed, including volunteers. Eventually the patients were stabilized and sent to surgery for attention to internal injuries and repair of broken bones and cuts.

In the eerie calm that typically settles over emergency rooms following events such as this, I noticed Maggie, the new candystriper, sitting limply on a stool in a corner. She was staring into space, gray as a ghost.

"Are you O.K.?" I asked. Forlorn, Maggie looked up in response; she tried to speak but could not. No reply was needed; she was about to be sick. Afterward, the nurses bedded her down on an empty stretcher for a few moments, and she felt better.

"Your first time in the E.R.?" I inquired.

"Pretty obvious, isn't it?" Maggie was not proud of her performance.

"Now you're a pro. The next time will be easy. By the way, why on earth did you volunteer for all this glamour?"

"Don't laugh, but I wanted to date medical students. I thought this would be a good way to meet them."

Maggie proved to be a regular in the E.R. She continued her volunteer work while in graduate school. On one occasion I jokingly asked her whether her original plan—to date medical students—had been successful.

"Fortunately not!" she said, laughing. "That's not the point anymore: I've been married for over a year."

"Then what is the point? Why do you still volunteer? You can't be hooked on the candystripe fashions."

"This may sound irrational," she replied, "but I feel more complete when I work here. Strangely, when the work is hardest—even when it's gruesome—I feel the best. During the summer, when I'm away, I miss this crazy place!"

Maggie's experience occurred long before the helper's high was described. It is a classic example of nature's built-in reward system to those who help others.

THE HEALER'S HIGH

An extreme form of altruism taking place hundreds of times every day in hospitals and emergency rooms is the resuscitation attempt. Resuscitation is an immensely demanding form of helping because there is no room for mistakes. A few seconds may mean the difference between survival and death. This is the ultimate challenge for every member of the health care team—nurse, physician, respiratory therapist, X-ray and electrocardiogram technician, and others. To be effective, actions must flow in a smooth, coordinated way, and the various members of the treatment team must function as a single unit. Each action must be guided by intelligence, and yet, because there is little time to think and reason, everything must be done with reflex rapidity.

Having participated as a physician in hundreds of these events through the years, I am convinced that something akin to the helper's high—what might be called the "healer's high"—affects many of the people involved during and after the resuscitation. This feeling can only be described as an altered state of awareness—an exalted feeling that there is an unqualified, exquisite rightness to things. This feeling does not depend on whether the resuscitation is successful; it is there whether or not the patient lives.

When resuscitations work best, each team member seems actually to know what the others are thinking. The nurse "reads the mind" of the physician in charge, knows which cardiac injection is needed next, and hands it to him or her even before it is asked for; someone intuitively knows that the person giving cardiac compression is tiring and rushes to relieve him or her before any words are exchanged. As a result, a heady feeling of closeness and unity can pervade the entire resuscitation team.

This can happen optimally only if there is a true forgetting of self during resuscitation attempts. But why during resuscitation? Perhaps because the egoistic self perceives the gravity of the situation and retires momentarily from its customary domination of consciousness. It quits the stage—and as it does so, the felt result frequently is the healer's high.

Some physicians and nurses are simply not suited to emergency situations. They dread participating in resuscitations, and they usually manage to choose areas within health care that effectively shield them from these involvements. Some physicians cannot "go with the flow" that is required in the resuscitation attempt. They may behave in ways that magnify the egoistic self, with bravado or tempestuous behavior—yelling and screaming orders to nurses and technicians, wasting critical time in criticizing other team members, or throwing instruments around the room like a child having a tantrum. If the resuscitation is not successful, they may blame someone else—anything to keep the ego intact.

Others relish these events and seem to thrive on them. They take to resuscitations and crises with an innate naturalness, ease, and grace. What is the difference between these two groups? Why do many nurses make a career out of E.R. nursing, with its endless stream of bloody, broken bodies, unpredictable crises, resuscitation attempts, and death?

I have made a habit through the years of asking emergency room nurses why they continue to work in the E.R. The commonest answers are "It gets in your blood" and "I've done it for so long I can't leave it." But what does this mean? Could it be that these nurses develop an affinity for the healer's high and the calm that follows? Does the emergency room setting give them a periodic opportunity to shed the sense of the "small self" and participate in a larger, collective identity extending beyond the person? If this speculation is correct, then these dedicated E.R. nurses have transformed their healing efforts into a true spiritual path of self-discovery and personal growth, all without realizing it.

Occasionally things happen in the highly charged atmosphere surrounding resuscitations that seem utterly unexplainable except by supposing that there is indeed a collective mind enveloping all those who are present.

A sixty-year-old woman had collapsed at home and was rushed, unconscious and unresponsive, to the emergency room. Despite a lengthy

resuscitation attempt, all measures failed and finally were abandoned. The woman's pupils were dilated and fixed; she had no pulse or blood pressure; and the heart monitor on the wall recorded only a straight line. The patient was dead. Then the head nurse tidied up the woman, made the room presentable, and went to the waiting room to ask if the daughter wished to see her mother one last time. Heartbroken and crying, standing by her mother's side, she leaned to kiss her. Wiping her tears, she told her, "We love you, Mother, and we did our best to save you, but now we're going to have to let you go. Good-bye, Mother!" The daughter gave a final kiss and stepped to the door. There she turned once again toward her mother and a remarkable event happened. The right arm of the dead woman rose slowly, bending from the elbow, and waved good-bye.

ALTRUISM: DELAYED AND DISTANT EFFECTS

One of the most famous altruists of this century is Mother Teresa, the Catholic nun awarded a Nobel Peace Prize for her work with the poor in Calcutta. At Harvard University, psychologist David McClelland, mentioned above, showed a film about Mother Teresa to students, and measured the amount of IgA in their saliva before and after showing the film to see whether an increase occurred.[5] (Salivary IgA is an antibody that protects against colds and upper respiratory infections.) Some students said they liked the film of Mother Teresa going about her work, and in them IgA levels increased. But, interestingly, "even those who professed intense dislike for Mother Teresa—some said she was a fake and that her work did no good—showed immune function improvement."[6] McClelland believes this study shows how unconscious beliefs and motives affect people's bodily reactions more profoundly than ordinary awareness. He states that someone like Mother Teresa reaches "the consciously disapproving people in a part of their brains that they were unaware of and that was still responding to the strength of her tender loving care."[7]

When McClelland tested this study's validity by having the students watch a film on Attila the Hun, salivary IgA levels fell.

Altruism behaves like a miracle drug, and a strange one at that. It has beneficial effects on the person doing the helping—the helper's high; it benefits the person to whom the help is directed; and it can stimulate healthy responses in persons at a distance who may view it only obliquely.

Although studies on altruism and the helper's high sometimes employ the complex language of neurotransmitters, receptor sites, and chemicals such as the endorphins, these behaviors are really not esoteric. Everyone knows it feels good to "do something nice" for someone else. Part of the warm feeling may well be due to coming home—returning to our original, undivided, larger Self, the part of us that connects, that knows no divisions in space and time.

Healing at a Distance:
Era III Medicine

THE POWER OF PRAYER

> We tend to think that the purpose of prayer is to
> terminate sickness, but we forget that the purpose of
> sickness may be to initiate prayer, or, more gener-
> ally, a consciousness of the infinite.
>
> —BRAD LEMLEY[1]

We will now take seriously the possibility that we and all other
persons are indeed, at some level of the psyche, part of a larger Self
that is boundless. If so, this would imply that we are potentially
capable of contacting those who are far removed from us, but with
whom we are in some sense connected. But in addition to contacting
them, can we do more?

The questions we now examine are: can we use our efforts to
assist healing in those who are distant from us? and if so, what is the
evidence?

My first patient as an eager, third-year medical student, fresh from two
years in the classroom, was a "70-year-old black male with terminal lung
cancer." My assignment involved taking a detailed history, performing a

physical examination, and presenting the case the following day to the interns, residents, and attending faculty members.

At my first opportunity I went to the patient's four-bed room, but on opening the door, I immediately stopped short. The curtain was drawn tightly around the bed for privacy. All I could see, from the knees downward, were the legs of a very large group of people ringing the bed. I watched the feet as they stamped in unison below the curtain— first one foot, then the other. In a booming, deep voice the leader of the crowd would shout words I could not understand, followed by the chorus's sonorous chant. Finally the chanting stopped and the leader began to pray for the recovery of the patient.

I was intimidated. Although I had grown up in a culture that honored prayer, the entreaties to the Almighty I was accustomed to were more "polite"—voiced in church, around the dinner table, or in private. I had never seen prayers advanced in public in such a brazen fashion. Clutching my small black bag and wearing my short white coat, the hallmark of the third-year student, I slunk silently out of the room, hoping to return at a more opportune moment.

Later I completed my assignment and presented the case the next day at the clinical conference. No doubt about it: the old man was hopeless. The lung cancer had been proven by biopsy to be an aggressive, highly malignant type, for which no satisfactory treatment existed. When the meager treatment alternatives were explained to him, he declined them and decided to leave the hospital. The consensus was uniform: his fate was sealed; he would be dead in a matter of weeks.

A year later the old man returned to the hospital and was admitted for a completely unrelated reason. This time a different student, a friend of mine, was assigned to his case. Reviewing his past records, he came across my name in the notes of the previous hospitalization. That night he called me on the phone and told me that my "terminal" patient of a year ago had surfaced. I could not believe it.

The next day I went to the radiology department and reviewed all his chest X rays, comparing the picture of a year ago to his current one. The change was striking: where there once was a dense, infiltrating cancer, healthy lung tissue now existed. The radiologist's interpretation read in part: ". . . there has been a striking response to the intercurrent treatment, with no present evidence of the previously existing carcinoma." The only hitch was that *there had been no intercurrent treatment.*

I contacted the resident physician who had assigned me the case a year ago and asked his opinion. He was not troubled in the least by this turn of events.

"We see this," he replied. "It's just 'the natural course of the disease.' Sometimes cancers take unexpected turns. Who knows?—maybe the biopsy was wrong."

I tracked down the patient the next day and inquired about what had happened. For him there was no mystery. His minister and friends had prayed for him, and now he was cured: it was as simple as that.

"Why, Doctor" he said respectfully, "is that so hard to understand?"

> Why is it when we talk to God we are said to be praying, and when God talks to us we're said to be schizophrenic?
>
> —LILY TOMLIN

Sir Francis Chichester (1901–1972) was one of the greatest adventurers of the twentieth century. In his early days he was a pioneer in aviation, the first person to fly alone from New Zealand to Australia, and from Australia to Japan—a feat he accomplished in a plane weighing less than 900 pounds. Chichester was too old to be accepted as a flying officer in World War II, but he taught navigation to RAF pilots and logged more flying time than many active pilots. After the war he took up sailing, achieving worldwide fame for sailing around the world in his thirty-nine-foot boat, *Gypsy Moth*. Prior to this feat, however, he made two solo trips across the Atlantic from England to New York in 1960 and 1962.

It is not generally known that in 1959, before his initial transatlantic voyage, Chichester nearly died from lung cancer. His diagnosis seems beyond doubt, having been established by numerous studies including a lung biopsy taken through a bronchoscope, an inflexible tube inserted deep into the airways. Five different doctors—surgeons, radiologists, and physicians including a lung specialist—agreed on the diagnosis and

informed him his only chance was the complete removal of one lung. With
the advise and support of Sheila, his courageous wife, he refused
surgery. It almost proved his undoing. As he described his ordeal of
many months:

> "Hospital routine; dreadful nights, lying for hour after hour
> unable to sleep, sometimes choking and gasping for
> breath. . . . I developed a terrified dread of that slow
> choking within. I despised myself as I became an abject coward
> about dying that way. As each fresh crisis built up, I wanted to
> cry as if surrendering to that weakness would give me respite."

Chichester's condition deteriorated, and one night everyone gave up
hope for him. He survived the night, but thereafter could breathe only
propped up on one elbow. Since he had refused surgery, his physicians,
apparently in a last-ditch effort, treated him with antibiotic pills, which
he distrusted and hid. Suddenly Chichester experienced a "tremendous
urge" to go to the south of France. He checked into a hotel in St. Paul
de Vence, bought some oxygen to help him stay alive, found an
iconoclastic doctor, became a vegetarian, and fasted periodically.
Chichester's cancer went away. In the end he attributed his cure largely
to his wife and the power of prayer:

> "[Sheila] has a strange and amazing flair for health and
> healing. She believes most strongly in the power of prayer.
> When I was at my worst, she rallied many people to pray for
> me, my friends and others. Whether Protestants, Roman
> Catholics, or Christian Scientists, she rallied them indefatigably
> to prayer. I feel shy about my troubles being imposed on
> others, but the power of prayer is miraculous."

One year later Chichester won the first east-to-west race across the
Atlantic since 1870, sailing his small craft three thousand miles in 40 ½
days—and he repeated the feat just two years later in a record-breaking
33 days, 15 hours.[2]

In the world of medical science, isolated examples such as the two
"prayer cases" here are not considered convincing. The old adage
"Beware the series of one!" expresses the researcher's inherent

suspicion of anecdotal cases. In assessing the effect of prayer, the question always to be asked is: When comparable groups of patients are studied in a well-designed experiment, with only one group being prayed for, is there a difference in the outcome of the two groups?

Dr. Randolph Byrd, a cardiologist and faculty member of the University of California Medical School at San Francisco, studied almost four hundred patients who were admitted to the coronary care unit of San Francisco General Hospital. Most of the patients had had or were suspected of having had a heart attack. They were divided roughly into two groups. Both received state-of-the-art medical care; however, one group was prayed for as well. Their first names and brief sketches of their condition were given to various Protestant and Catholic prayer groups throughout the United States, who were asked to pray for them. This was a double-blind study, meaning that neither the nurses, physicians, nor patients knew who was and was not being prayed for. This meant that preferential care could not unconsciously be given by the health care professionals to one group; nor could the prayed-for group "try harder" to get well, knowing they were being prayed for. Neither was one group sicker than the other; there were no statistical differences in the severity of illness between the two groups.

When this meticulous study was over, the prayed-for group appeared to have been given some "miracle drug." They did better clinically in several ways:

1. They were far less likely to develop congestive heart failure, a condition in which the lungs fill with fluid as a consequence of the failure of the heart to pump properly (eight compared to twenty patients).

2. They were five times less likely to require antibiotics (three compared to sixteen patients), and three times less likely to need diuretics (five compared to fifteen patients).

3. None of the prayed-for group required endotracheal intubation, in which an artificial "breathing tube" is inserted in the throat and attached to a mechanical ventilator, while twelve of the other group required mechanical ventilatory support.

4. Fewer of the prayed-for group developed pneumonia (three compared to thirteen).

5. Fewer of those prayed for experienced cardiopulmonary arrest requiring resuscitation (CPR; three compared to fourteen).

6. None of the prayed-for group died, compared to three deaths among those not prayed for (this difference was not statistically significant).[3]

The outcome of this meticulous clinical experiment was so striking that it aroused national interest. If the therapy being evaluated had been a new drug or surgical procedure, it would undoubtedly have been heralded as a medical breakthrough. Even a noted skeptic of "psychic healing," Dr. William Nolen, author of *The Making of a Surgeon,* remarked that perhaps physicians should be writing in their orders, "Pray for my patient three times a day."

A striking aspect of this study is that it violates one of the most hallowed assumptions of modern medicine: that the therapist, physician, or healer must be on site. Nothing in modern science indicates that "distant healing" can occur. This experiment also challenges the equally engrained belief that when the mind plays a role in recovery, it is necessarily the mind of the patient. It has been assumed that one's thoughts may affect one's own body, as a multitude of data show, but not the body of someone else. Yet another striking feature of the study is that the effects of prayer did not depend on the awareness of the recipient, since no one knew who was receiving prayer.

This experiment does not stand alone. For a decade the Spindrift organization in Salem, Oregon, has studied scientifically the ability of praying persons to affect the behavior of simple biological systems— for example, the germination rate of seeds or the metabolic activity of yeast cultures. Their experiments are elegant, quantitative, and repeatable. Like the coronary care unit study, these experiments suggest that prayer exerts a powerful effect that can be readily measured.[4]

NONCONTACT THERAPEUTIC TOUCH

From ancient times to the present, people have claimed the ability to heal from a distance and the ability to heal by "laying on of hands," in which actual physical contact takes place. These two healing techniques have recently been hybridized through the landmark research of nursing academician Dolores Krieger of New York University.[5] In what is called therapeutic touch, the healer's hands do not actually touch the patient but are held a short distance from the patient's body.

To evaluate whether or not healing can take place when the hands are held a short distance from the body without physical contact, and without the patient being aware of any healing intent, researcher Daniel P. Wirth performed a double-blind study involving forty-four patients with artificially created, full-skin-thickness surgical wounds. The subjects would, for five minutes at a time, insert their arm with the wound through a circular hole cut out in a wall beyond which they could not see. They were falsely told that the purpose of this procedure was to measure "biopotentials" from the surgical wound site with a noncontact device. A noncontact therapeutic touch practitioner was present in the adjoining room only during sessions for the twenty-three patients of the active treatment group; the room was vacant during the sessions for the remaining twenty-one patients. As the practitioner attempted to heal the wounds, she meticulously avoided any physical contact with the subjects. At several stages each wound was measured for healing by a physician who was unaware of the group to which the patient belonged.

Importantly, since the subjects had no idea they were participating did not *believe* they were receiving a healing treatment, and since they received neither overt nor covert suggestions of being participants in a healing experiment, the placebo response, suggestion, expectation, or belief cannot be held responsible for the healing that occurred.

The results were highly significant statistically in many ways. By the eighth day, the wound sizes of the treated subjects showed much less variation than those of the untreated subjects, and were significantly smaller. This was also true on the sixteenth day, when in addition, thirteen of the twenty-three treated subjects were completely healed (wound size zero), compared with *none* of the untreated group. This study indicated that noncontact therapeutic touch is an effective method of healing wounds, even if the subject is unaware of its occurrence.[6]

Wirth's study is buttressed by much previous experimental evidence for the effectiveness of noncontact therapeutic touch, almost all of which has come from the field of nursing. In addition to the work of Krieger mentioned above, the pioneering work of nurse-academician Janet Quinn has been invaluable in demonstrating scientifically the beneficial effects of this technique.[7]

How does noncontact therapeutic touch work? Is there some subtle exchange of energy between healer and patient? Researcher John T. Zimmerman, of the Bio-Electro-Magnetics Institute, believes so. He has studied the electromagnetic energy fields that may be involved in this form of therapy using a superconducting quantum interference device or SQUID. When he studied three separate healers, signals several hundred times higher than background noise appeared during four out of seven healing attempts. But when nonhealers were tested, there was no signal at all. Zimmerman cites studies performed at the Jiao Tong University in Shanghai on a gifted Chinese healer who used the ancient qi gong method of healing. Qi gong, also a noncontact technique, postulates a subtle form of energy, or *chi,* which is utilized by the healer. The Shanghai studies suggested that electromagnetic energy in the near-infrared range is emitted from the healer's palms during healing work. Zimmerman hypothesizes that infrared and microwave electromagnetic radiation from the hands actually does the healing work.[8]

THE HEALING OF SOCIETIES

Some of the most striking evidence that minds can exert healing power at a distance comes from recent research in Transcendental Meditation. Moreover, this research suggests that not only individuals but entire population centers and countries can be healed in significant ways. One study reported the effects of a meditating group in Jerusalem in 1983. There was an inverse correlation between the size of the meditating group and war deaths and war intensity in neighboring Lebanon, as well as crimes and violence in Israel. Analysis showed that changes in group size preceded the events being measured, supporting a causal interpretation. The number of war deaths decreased 70 percent on days when meditation attendance was high compared with when it was low.[9] In addition, a similar study showed an inverse relationship between the size of a meditating group and the level of violent crime in the Washington, D.C. area.[10] There is a suggestion that meditators may actually create changes in brain chemistry in those around them. In one particular study, when large numbers of meditators gathered to meditate, nonmeditators in the surrounding town showed evidence of an increased rate of metabolism for serotonin, an important brain chemical. Since low levels of serotonin have been associated with high levels of aggressiveness, the higher turnover rate suggests a chemical correlate in the brain to the peaceful, calming social changes seen in earlier studies. This puts the social changes on firmer footing and suggests they are not just statistical anomalies, as skeptics have claimed.[11]

As a result of these intriguing findings, several researchers working in this area, including physicists, have proposed that consciousness is a genuinely "nonlocal" field, which is not confined to points in space and time.[12] This would mean that consciousness would not be limited to individual brains or bodies or to the present moment, but would have infinite extension.

Some of the evidence favoring a nonlocal view of the mind is hardly exotic; it deals with the behavior of the physical brain itself. Experiments using the electroencephalogram (EEG), a measure of the electrophysiological activity in the brain, show that distant, direct communication from person to person can occur without sensory cues—that is, without verbalization, visualization, or physical contact. Researchers Jacobo Grinberg-Zylberbaum and Julieta Ramos of the Universidad Nacional Autónoma of Mexico studied paired subjects in a soundproof and darkened Faraday cage, a lead-screened chamber that filters out all outside electromagnetic activity. Each pair was instructed to close their eyes and to try to communicate by becoming aware of the other's presence and to signal the experimenter when they felt this had occurred. EEG analysis showed that during periods when the subjects reported communicating, the patterns of the hemispheres of each subject's brain were "very alike." At such times, there were also similarities between the EEG patterns of the separated subjects. One subject's EEG patterns became similar to those of each of three partners with whom he was paired. In one session, when the partners reported a feeling of having blended, their EEG patterns became virtually identical. Both before and after the experimental period, during control sessions when the subjects were not trying to communicate, the subjects showed no synchrony between their own hemispheres or between each other. Based on these findings, the researchers postulate the existence of "neuronal fields" that can interact and alter one another.[13]

These effects resemble what psychophysiologist Jeanne Achterberg, in her book *Imagery in Healing,* termed *transpersonal imagery,* which she defined as the ability of the consciousness of one person to affect the physical body of another.[14] At the Mind Science Foundation in San Antonio, Texas, researchers William Braud and Marilyn Schlitz put nonlocal, transpersonal imagery to a test. They examined whether people could use specific mental imagery to change the physical reactions of someone distant with whom they had no physical or sensory contact. Thirteen experiments were done using this strategy. A significant relationship was found between a person's use of calming or activating imagery and the electrodermal activity of another isolated, distant subject (electrodermal activity is an indicator of physiological arousal). "The findings," the researchers stated, "demonstrate reliable and relatively robust anomalous interactions between living systems at a distance."[15]

DIAGNOSIS AT A DISTANCE

Not only can the consciousness of persons be used *therapeutically* for others, it can be used *diagnostically* as well. Perhaps the most persuasive example of this phenomenon is described in a recent book, *The Creation of Health: Merging Traditional Medicine with Intuitive Diagnosis,* by C. Norman Shealy and Caroline M. Myss.[16]

In 1985 Dr. Shealy, formerly a Harvard-based neurosurgeon and researcher who founded the American Holistic Medical Association, met and began to work with Caroline Myss. Previously a journalist who had begun to work in publishing, Myss had no formal training in medicine or health. She knew, however, that since early childhood she had the innate ability to know things intuitively. Dr. Shealy asked her to put her intuitive skills to work in diagnosing illness in his patients. While his patient was with him in his office in Missouri, he would phone Myss in New Hampshire, 1,200 miles away. Initially he would simply give her his patient's name and birthdate, and she would then tell him her impressions. Most of these dealt with the patient's psychological conflicts. But as their partnership evolved, Shealy encouraged her to be as specific as possible about physical abnormalities. Then Myss began intuitively "entering" the patient's body and speaking as if she were the actual patient. Shealy encouraged her to travel through the patient's body systematically, examining the relative health of each organ system. Shealy: "Just how good is Caroline? [The data show] she is 93% accurate. [Such accuracy] is a fantastic accomplishment." This is, in fact, an understatement. Even with sophisticated diagnostic tools such as blood analyses and X rays, medical diagnosticians seldom achieve these levels in the earliest phase of diagnosis. The spatial separation between Myss and the patient is apparently totally overcome in the intuitive process. For her, the impersonal situation that results from this distancing is an important key to her success, because it permits her to "receive information that a more personal connection would otherwise tend to block."

Interestingly, Myss was hesitant to become involved with intuitive diagnosis. She had always considered her talent a curiosity, something she could casually employ at will. She was particularly leary of labels such as "psychic" and was concerned about being thought fraudulent or a "crackpot."

Fifty examples of Myss's intuitive diagnoses are presented in Shealey's and her book. Most of them correspond to Shealey's actual medical diagnosis with great accuracy. For instance, when Myss's diagnosis was "migraine headache, myofascial pain," Shealy's diagnosis also was "migraine headache, myofascial pain." Her "chest pain due to trauma" corresponded to his "post-surgical chest pain, left." Her "malignancy of [the] brain" was his "metastatic brain cancer." Shealy's estimation of Myss's skills is unequivocal: "I have not seen anyone more accurate than Caroline," he says. "Not even a physician!"

ERA III MEDICINE

How do the above phenomena—prayer, noncontact therapeutic touch, extended effects of meditation, effects of transpersonal or distant imagery, and diagnosis at a distance—fit into modern medicine? *Can* they fit? I believe the answer is yes, if we are bold enough to extend our views of the mind.

Looking back on the history of medicine since the dawn of the scientific era, it is possible to discern three distinct types of healing methodologies. Since these fall into a kind of historical sequence, they can be referred to as eras.

Era I may be called "mechanical," "materialistic," or "physical" medicine. It encompasses the therapies that are largely favored in the West today and that have dominated our approach to healing for at least one hundred years, including the use of surgery, drugs, and irradiation. Era I medicine is guided by the classical laws of matter and energy described in the seventeenth century by Sir Isaac Newton. According to this perspective the entire universe, including the body, is a vast clockwork that functions according to deterministic principles. All forms of therapy, to be effective, must be "physical." In Era I, therefore, the effects of mind and consciousness are considered of secondary importance if they are considered at all.

Era I medicine is a majestic achievement in the history of healing. Its accomplishments speak for themselves and are too numerous to name. These achievements are so significant that most persons believe the future of medicine still lies solidly in Era I approaches.

Approximately four decades ago, however, another unique period in the history of healing began solidly to take shape—Era II or "mind-body" medicine. Although mind-body approaches have been around since antiquity, at long last they began to be studied scientifically. It became possible to show that perceptions, emotions, attitudes, thoughts, and perceived meanings affect the body, sometimes in dramatic, life-or-death ways as illustrated by the tales in this book. All the major diseases of our day—heart disease, hypertension, cancer, and more—have by now been shown to be influenced, at least to some degree, by the mind.

The hallmark of Era II is the intimate connection between the mind, brain, and the various organs of the body. Candace B. Pert, former chief of brain chemistry at the National Institute of Mental Health, has expressed unequivocally this intimate association. As quoted earlier, she states that we can no longer sharply distinguish between the brain and the body and need to start looking at how consciousness can be projected into the parts of the body.

A variety of therapies have arisen to take advantage of these connections. Biofeedback, meditation, relaxation therapies, and a host of other techniques that employ imagery are today quite common. They do not conflict with Era I therapies, but exist side by side with them in a complementary relationship. Sometimes Era I and Era II approaches have fused, leading to entirely new disciplines such as the developing field of psychoneuroimmunology, which recognizes a functional unity between the psyche and the neurological and immune systems.

The major difference between Eras I and II is that the latter attributes a causal power to the mind. Still the two have much in common. With respect to the mind, they are both *local* in emphasis—which means they consider the mind to be localized to points in space (the brain and body) and time (the present moment). This is most obvious in Era I, in which the mind is considered by most bioscientists to be a byproduct or epiphenomenon of the brain that somehow emerged at a certain stage of chemical complexity in the evolution of living organisms. But Era II is also a local approach, because it emphasizes the mind and consciousness of the *individual* person operating on the *individual* body—all within the classical framework of Era I. In addition, most researchers working in Era II medicine seem to believe that the mind is only a function of the chemistry and anatomy of the brain. Thus, in both Eras I and II, mind equals brain.

Many enthusiasts of Era II believe that the mind–body approaches that emphasize the action of one's mind on one's body are the ultimate form of therapy and that healing can go no "higher." But, as important an advance as Era II medicine has been, we can now see that it, like Era I healing, is also limited and incomplete. There are too many phenomena for which it cannot account, too many healing events left unexplainable, such as those reviewed above. In order to

MEDICAL ERAS*

	ERA I	ERA II	ERA III
SPACE-TIME CHARACTER-ISTIC	Local	Local	Nonlocal
SYNONYM	Mechanical, material, or physical medicine	Mind-body, complementary, or alternative medicine	Nonlocal medicine
DESCRIPTION	Causal, deterministic, describable by classical concepts of space-time and matter-energy. Mind not a factor; "mind" a result of brain mechanisms.	Mind a major factor in healing *within* the single person. Mind has causal power; is thus not fully explainable by classical concepts in physics. Includes but goes beyond Era I.	Mind a factor in healing both *within* and *between* persons. Mind not completely localized to points in space (brains or bodies) or time (present moment or single lifetimes). Mind is unbounded in space and time and thus ultimately unitary or one. Healing at a distance is possible. Not describable by classical concepts of space-time or matter-energy.
EXAMPLES	Any form of therapy focusing solely on effects of *things* on the body are Era I approaches—including techniques such as acupuncture and homeopathy, the use of herbs, etc. Almost all forms of "modern" medicine—drugs, surgery, irradiation, CPR, etc.—are included.	Any therapy emphasizing the effects of consciousness *solely* within the individual body is an Era II approach. Psycho-neuroimmunology, counseling, hypnosis, biofeedback, relaxation therapies, and most types of imagery-based "alternative" therapies are included.	Any therapy in which effects of consciousness bridge between different persons is an Era III approach. All forms of distant healing, intercessory prayer, "psychic" and shamanic healing, "miracles," diagnosis at a distance, and noncontact therapeutic touch are included.

*Copyright Larry Dossey, M.D. For a detailed description of the three medical eras, see my *Recovering the Soul* (New York: Bantam, 1989).

encompass these, we must postulate another era—Era III medicine.

Era III is a genuinely *nonlocal* approach to healing—it views the mind as unbounded, unconfined to points in space and time such as brains, bodies, or the present. Like Era II, Era III emphasizes the causal power of consciousness. But unlike Era II, it does not regard the mind as originating from the brain, although the mind is acknowledged to work through the brain. An additional unique feature of Era III is the ultimately unitary nature of the mind, which is a consequence of its unboundedness. (A detailed defense for these robust claims is given in my book *Recovering the Soul*.[17]) In the Era III view, then, minds are considered as omnipresent, infinite, immortal, and ultimately one. As a result, healing events that involve the mind may bridge persons who are widely separated from each other with no known sensory contact, and may do so instantly.

It is important to realize that Era III medicine goes beyond today's physics, because almost all physicists continue completely to ascribe all the manifestations of consciousness to the physical processes within the brain. Era III medicine denies that this is a complete explanation. Although it acknowledges that mental *content* and *levels* of awareness can be influenced by physical processes occurring in the brain and body, it ascribes a primary, causal efficacy to the mind because of the evidence suggesting the mind can do things that the brain cannot—such as acting across distances to facilitate healing, as in the prayer study of Byrd, or gaining information remotely, as in the distant diagnosis of Myss. In Era III, then, mind, not matter, is ultimately considered primary. As philosopher Willis Harman puts it, consciousness—not matter—was here first.

It is important to recognize that Era III medicine does not discard the majestic achievements of Eras I and II but, rather, honors them and includes them in a complementary way. Like Carol, whose story we saw in Chapter 1, many people do not understand this. Once they discover the therapeutic potential of the mind, therapy for them becomes "all mind." They may react with horror to Era I therapies, as if employing anything other than the mind in getting well were an ethical or moral compromise. But the Era III "medicine of nonlocality" recognizes that the approaches of Eras I and II still apply in certain situations and can be extraordinarily valuable.

I have discussed with dozens of groups the scientific evidence that has emerged from Era III–type therapeutic and diagnostic studies like those reviewed here. When many people learn about this evidence, they sense a genuine breakthrough in their beliefs about their health. Different people describe this breakthrough differently. Some speak of a sense of empowerment and validation, saying that "I always *believed* these methods worked, but I was unaware that there was solid evidence behind them." Others describe a decrease in their concern about their health. One woman, recovering from a serious illness, began to weep on hearing some of these studies. "I always thought getting well was entirely up to me and my doctor," she said. "This has always felt lonely and a terrible burden. Now I realize others can help. I know now I'm not alone."

The Place of Emptiness:
The Return of Miracles

As to me, I know of nothing else but miracles.

—WALT WHITMAN

The beauty of it is that we have to content ourselves with the recognition of the *miracle,* beyond which there is no legitimate way out.

—ALBERT EINSTEIN

The world has signed a pact with the devil; it had to. . . . The terms are clear: if you want to live, you have to die; you cannot have mountains and creeks without space, and space is a beauty married to a blind man. The blind man is Freedom, or Time, and he does not go anywhere without his great dog Death. The world came into being with the signing of the contract.

—ANNIE DILLARD
Pilgrim at Tinker Creek

Alvar Núñez Cabeza de Vaca, the great Spanish explorer who lived during the first half of the sixteenth century, followed the wake of Columbus to the new world. After becoming shipwrecked on the Texas coast, de Vaca feared murder by hostile natives. He took refuge where he could find it, including a pit in the harsh Texas territory where he spent several winter nights sleeping naked under a north wind. At that point de Vaca had lost everything. Yet he survived, and then he discovered that a most amazing thing had happened: he had the power to heal. Thus as he walked westward he would heal sick native people along the way. His fame spread ahead of him. Eventually he made his way back to Mexico and became once again a civilized Spaniard. At this point the events seemed to reverse themselves. Drawing closer to civilization, he lost not only the ability to heal, but the will to heal as well. The reason? As he said, there were "real doctors" in the city, and as he drew nearer to them he began to doubt his own healing powers.[1]

De Vaca's ability to heal was preceded by profound emptiness, a shipwreck of both body and spirit, a dark night of the soul in which he did not know he would survive. Out of this state a miracle was born.

Nearly five centuries after de Vaca buried himself in order to survive, a similar event took place in one of the most hostile regions on earth: the Antarctic continent. In July 1989, six men, each from a different nation, began the first unmechanized trek across Antarctica. This remarkable effort, known as the International Trans-Antarctica Expedition, was led by former science teacher Will Steger of the United States, who had led an expedition without resupply to the North Pole in 1986. For 220 days the group braved the worst weather in the world, enduring two months of storms, winds up to 90 miles an hour, and temperatures as low as −43° F. With only dogsleds and skis, following the longest and most difficult route across Antarctica, they completed their goal by traveling 3,741 miles.

Just two days before the completion of their journey a blinding snowstorm arose. At 4:30 in the afternoon, thirty-two-year-old Keizo Funatsu from Japan, the youngest member of the expedition and the team's expert with sled dogs, walked a few yards from the camp in the blizzard to feed the huskies. Although the men as always in such conditions had staked skis and poles every few yards between their tents, Keizo lost his way. Realizing his precarious situation, he took immediate measures for survival. Here is how he described the experience in his journal:

> Once I was in my snow ditch, blowing snow covered me in five, ten seconds. . . . I could breathe through a cavity close to my body, but the snow was blowing inside my clothes, and I was getting wet. I knew my teammates would be looking for me. I believed I would be found; it was just a matter of time. I had to believe that. . . .
>
> Very few people have that kind of experience, lost in the blizzard. I said to myself, 'Settle down, try and enjoy this.' In my snow ditch I truly felt Antarctica. With the snow and quiet covering me, I felt like I was in my mother's womb. I could hear my heart beat—boom, boom, boom—like a small baby's. My life seemed very small compared to nature, to Antarctica.

Two hours after Keizo lost his way in the whiteout conditions, the other team members discovered his absence and began a search, which had to be abandoned after four hours because of darkness and the storm. At 4:00 A.M. the next day they resumed. At 6:00 A.M. Keizo, unhurt, heard the searchers calling his name. He emerged from his snowy burial and stood up, shouting, "I am alive! I am alive!" Tears of joy flowed. Expedition leader Steger summed up the experience: "Finding Keizo alive was the greatest relief I have ever known."[2]

Completely covered with snow, Keizo Funatsu had realized that to do *anything* would have meant almost certain death. He had simply to be, not do. The images that flooded his mind were those of the most profound period of not-doing for anyone—being a baby in his mother's womb. Thus, buried alive at the bottom of the world, he could only wait patiently to see what the universe would deliver. His "being strategy" paid off with survival, as it did for de Vaca.

There is an aspect of experiences such as those of Cabeza de Vaca and Keizo Funatsu that runs counter to the modern belief that real change requires robust effort. In their extremity they really were not in control of what was occurring, and they were not actively *doing* something. Theirs was rather an attitude of watching, waiting, silence, and emptiness—ways of *being*, not doing.

Many persons who experience sudden breakthroughs in health— sudden improvements in the course of an illness that were not anticipated—describe something similar. They frequently speak of an inner attitude of accepting the universe on its own terms—not dictating what ought or should happen—in spite of the dreadful circumstances they are enduring at the time. They do not expend energy on being bitter, resentful, and angry for the hand they have been dealt. This is not a self-effacing, passive, giving-up stance; it is one of attunement and alignment with what they perceive to be the inherent rightness of all that is. A sense of empowerment and freedom frequently flows from this state, regardless of what may happen to the course of the illness. Pulitzer Prize–winning poet Gary Snyder has described this attitude of taking on the world as it is: "To be truly free one must take on the basic conditions as they are: painful, impermanent, and imperfect; and then be grateful, for in a fixed universe there would be no freedom."[3]

The message being delivered today to many sick persons is the opposite. They are told in endless books and seminars that only if they demonstrate an antagonistic, robust "fighting spirit" will they have a chance to "beat cancer" or recover from heart disease or some other malady. But there are other ways to "fight," as the experiences of Cabeza de Vaca and Keizo Funatsu tell us. These ways require giving up the hubristic, arrogant, and narcissistic belief that the universe revolves around our own condition and should invariably dance to our tune. They require that we cease dictating our own terms to the universe, that we hush our petulant little "I want it thus," that we stop our incessant efforts to beat the world into line. This cessation can ideally create a vacuum or an emptiness into which healing *can* flow.

Today patients are anything but empty. They are loaded down with expectations, directives, pills, and surgery, and an endless chain of advice from doctors, nurses, friends, and self-help experts. Even if nothing works they are often dispatched from the hospital pumped full of "hope"—the suggestion that a cure or breakthrough could be just around the corner. Patients are often bewildered in this thera-peutic flurry; they frequently go from aisle to aisle in the clinical supermarket, dazed, sampling a bit of everything—the orthodox and traditional, the "alternative," the "holistic."

Where does the drive to fill up every waking moment by *doing* something to improve our health come from? Researcher and author Lewis Thomas believes this urge has become endemic in our culture, and that it has some extremely negative consequences. He writes:

> Americans are obsessed with their health. [This has a] negative side: . . . the impression that we are constructed as a kind of imperfect organism—fallible and fragile and likely to collapse unless we are propped up by what it is now fashionable to call the health care system.
>
> There's an awful lot of talk these days implying that it is abnormal to be unhappy. You read things that suggest that if you're unhappy and if you're depressed, as everybody is from time to time, you are ill. There's a whole new profession of people who advise other people on how to live a life—as though you could take courses in some part of the university and learn how to live wisely and sagaciously and end up being happy or avoid being unhappy. This has been greatly overdone.
>
> There's a lot of genuine mental illness. . . . But it worries me that people, especially the young, are being brought up to believe that if they're unhappy, they ought to go see a counselor and get what's called guidance.[4]

One is reminded of a comment of Saint Teresa of Avila: "It is a great grace of God to practice self-examination; but too much is as bad as too little."

In the pervasive hubbub over "health care" it is almost impossible for patients to find an opportunity for emptiness. Yet for radical healing—for what has traditionally been called miraculous or "break-through" healing—to return and to work, emptiness has to be experienced. Occasionally people do experience emptiness, whether from exhaustion or insight. Unexpected healings seem most frequent in these persons. Perhaps it has always been so. The reports of the ill undergoing miraculous healings at famous shrines such as Lourdes reveal the same finding: the "empty" patient who is filled with gratitude and acceptance is most likely to be healed.

Modern physicians, like patients, also find emptiness an almost impossible state to achieve. They equate emptiness with passivity and backwardness. The imperative to act is so strong that in most circles it is considered an ethical weakness to stand by, wait, and do nothing.

The "empty healer" is not just a metaphor. Psychologist Lawrence LeShan has extensively studied many genuine "faith healers." The great majority of them describe a psychological state of emptiness that accompanies their work, as if they are a transmitter for some greater energy lying outside themselves. Many say they are only a conduit which cannot function if already filled.[5]

Today most people believe, like Cabeza de Vaca, that the real doctors are still in the city—at the hospitals, the academic institutions, the research facilities. Healing, most say, comes from surgery, drugs, *things*. Healing originating from a frill-less, gadgetless physician—an *empty* physician—is simply unthinkable, a contradiction in terms. But although nature may abhor a vacuum, healing *requires* it for miracles to occur. Miracles require learning once again to dwell in a place that has become foreign to the modern mind, the place of emptiness, the domain of being instead of doing. It means becoming sensitive once more to the movements of the universe, instead of trying always to move it ourselves.

Next we take a closer look at how the paradoxes of healing manifest in the actual experiences of sick persons—at how *being,* not just doing, sets the stage for the miraculous.

Standing in the Void:
Paradoxical and Rational Healing

Practice not-doing and everything will fall into place.

—LAO-TZU
Tao Te Ching

Nothing is more fatal to health than overcare of it.

—BENJAMIN FRANKLIN

If the world stands bewildered and confused in the face of its trouble, it is partly because we Westerners have made a God of activity; we have yet to learn how to *be,* as we have already learnt how to do.

—PAUL BRUNTON[1]

I am not eager, bold
Or strong—all that is past.
I am ready *not* to do,
At last, at last!

—SAINT PETER CANISIUS[2]
(1521–1597)

When we must deal with problems, we instinctively
resist trying the way that leads through obscurity
and darkness. We wish to hear only of unequivocal
results, and completely forget that these results can
only be brought about when we have ventured into,
and emerged again from, darkness.

—C. G. JUNG

A thirty-two-year-old man witnessed his father plan the murder of a
beloved relative, which was actually committed. Overwhelmed with fear
that he would be called to testify against his father, the man completely
repressed this knowledge into his unconscious mind. Around the time he
did so, he developed throat cancer. However, during an intense
psychotherapy session the night before he was scheduled to have the
growth removed surgically, he broke down and recounted the entire
event. With much crying and trembling, he relived the painful memories
and emotions. Within hours of doing so, he finished the first meal he was
able to eat without pain in weeks. And within four days, the tumor was
completely gone.

A fifty-two-year-old woman suffered from uterine cancer that had spread
to her intestine. She was expected to die within weeks. But when her
"much hated" husband died, she experienced a sudden, complete
recovery.

Writer Gregg Levoy, who reported the above cases, observes that the
breakthrough in healing experienced by these persons usually involves some dramatic personal and psychological catalyst—a recon-
ciliation with a long-despised father or mother, the birth of a
grandchild, a religious conversion, or the removal of obstacles to a
career. These people suddenly find life more meaningful, more
satisfying. They are no longer overwhelmed by hopelessness, guilt,
or anger. They have discovered a new way to *be*. Psychiatrist Charles
Weinstock, formerly director of New York's Psychosomatic Cancer
Study Group, agrees. Speaking of cases of spontaneous remission of
cancer he says, "In each there was a major, favorable change in the
patient's life situation just preceding the cancer shrinkage."[3]

It is important to understand that ways of being *are not opposed* to ways of doing. Cases of breakthrough healing abound in which the sick person employs both. In fact, these cases are probably more numerous than those in which only changes of being preceed the healing event. What is needed is a complementary "both-and" approach, not an "either-or" strategy.

Even in cases where the recovering person seems to rely almost solely on an action-oriented, doing approach, new ways of being are decisively involved if one looks closely at what is going on, as the following case shows.

> When Robert was in his twenties, his doctor told him he had three months to live. Robert had testicular cancer which had spread to his chest, lungs, and lymph nodes. One cancerous lump on his neck was so large it forced him to tilt his head almost to his shoulder. He received palliative cobalt radiation treatments for relief of pain and to keep the lumps from growing bigger. In spite of the essentially zero chance for survival that he was given, Robert decided to face his disease with a particular way of being—facing the grim prognosis with a fighting spirit. As he put it, "I wasn't going to curl up my toes and die."
>
> His new choice of how to be led to new ways of doing. He immediately began to take life-affirming, positive steps. These included deciding to marry his girlfriend and to become an Episcopal priest. (He had already finished his seminary studies but had been ambivalent about actually entering the priesthood.) Within a month of these decisions, he was both married and ordained.
>
> Robert also became what some would call a "bad patient." He argued and fought with his nurses and doctors, "insisting on explanations for everything they wanted to do, not accepting the lord-and-master routine." And he devised different ways of being not only toward his human health care providers but the nonhuman ones as well, such as the cobalt machine. "I collaborated with [it]," he said, "rooting it on, not being passive."
>
> The results were astonishing to Robert's physician. Within a month after Robert decided "to do things more appropriate to living than dying," X rays showed no trace of cancer in Robert's body.
>
> The response of those around him was interesting, almost amusing. "Everyone wanted to lay claim to being the healer," Robert stated. His

psychologist said it was the therapy that did the trick. The radiologist was sure it was the cobalt. His bishop explained everything through "divine grace."

Were the changes just a temporary lapse of the disease, a "spontaneous remission" soon to recur? Hardly. A decade later Robert completed his training as a psychologist, and thirty years later he is still cancer free.[4]

In some cases it appears that being—in the form of beliefs and meanings—is paramount, even when the person is certain that only doing is involved, as in the following famous case from the 1950s:

A man with an advanced cancer was no longer responding to radiation treatment. He was given a single injection of an experimental drug, Krebiozen, considered by some at the time to be a "miracle cure" (it has since been discredited). The results were shocking to the patient's physician, who stated that his tumors "melted like snowballs on a hot stove."

Later the man read studies suggesting the drug was ineffective, and his cancer began to spread once more. At this point his doctor, acting on a hunch, administered a placebo intravenously. The man was told the plain water was a "new, improved" form of Krebiozen. Again, his cancer shrank away dramatically. Then he read in the newspapers the American Medical Association's official pronouncement: Krebiozen was a worthless medication. The man's faith vanished, and he was dead within days.[5]

THE SPECTRUM OF HEALING:
THE PARADOXICAL AND THE RATIONAL

paradox: a statement seemingly absurd or contradictory, yet in fact true.[6]

"A paradox is truth standing on its head to attract attention."

—*The Paradoxicon*[7]

It is possible to arrange *all* healing activities or experiences in a hierarchy or spectrum, based on the relative degree of being and doing involved. Those healing strategies that employ a lot of doing seem reasonable to us; they make sense, and are explained by science; they seem rational. Because of this, "doing therapies" can be called *rational* forms of healing. "Being therapies" are different. Their results seem frequently to arise from nowhere without cause. They are decidedly not rational because they lack a scientific explanation. Science cannot explain, for example, how prayer could be effective at a distance, or how a deep clearing of emotion can lead to the disappearance of a cancer, as in cases discussed above. These events are shrouded in mystery. Because they lack a reasonable explanation we can call them *paradoxical*. We have, then, two major domains of healing events, the rational and the paradoxical, in which ways of doing and ways of being, respectively, are most important.

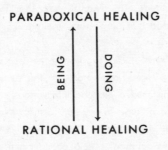

Figure 2.

Examples of rational healing are everywhere. They are largely made up of the Era I, physically based therapies noted earlier [see p. 191), such as surgery, medication, irradiation, exercise, and diet. In each of these approaches, science has explanations for why the techniques work. These approaches conform to our current views of the nature of matter, energy, and causation. But as we move up the spectrum of the therapies toward the domain of paradox, the conformity diminishes. The therapies in Figure 3, which have been arbitrarily chosen among the many approaches, make the point.

Consider psychological counseling. We use the word "break-through" to describe healing events in counseling or analysis. These life-changing events may occur out of the blue after years of counseling during which no progress was made. We cannot see

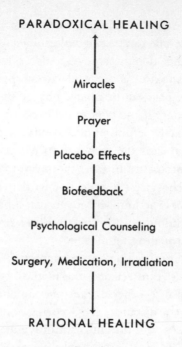

PARADOXICAL HEALING

↑

Miracles

|

Prayer

|

Placebo Effects

|

Biofeedback

|

Psychological Counseling

|

Surgery, Medication, Irradiation

|

↓

RATIONAL HEALING

Figure 3.

breakthroughs coming, they are utterly unpredictable, we do not know how to have another one on demand, and we do not know what caused them. As the Scottish psychiatrist R. D. Laing wrote in his book *The Divided Self:* "The really decisive moments in psychotherapy, as every patient or therapist who has ever experienced them knows, are unpredictable, unique, unforgettable, always unrepeatable, and often indescribable."[8] For all these reasons, a psychological breakthrough is paradoxical.

As we move up the list of therapies in Figure 3, the results of our efforts become even more difficult to predict. Consider biofeedback, in which electronic instruments are used to measure and "feed back" body information to the conscious mind, so that voluntary control can be gained over certain physical processes, like blood pressure, muscle tension, brain waves, and skin temperature. In the early phases of biofeedback training the person quickly discovers that one can only gain control and "make it happen" by letting go. Active effort only delays progress; "not doing" becomes the key to success. "Passive volition" is the phrase biofeedback therapists frequently use to describe this strategy. Although one makes the choice to *do* biofeedback therapy, one can't *make* the results happen. The paradox is that of doing by not doing, achieving success by not striving.

Even more paradoxical is the well-known placebo response, in which, for example, pain can be relieved by giving a pill that has no known biological effect if the person believes it is a potent medication. This response is by definition not rational, because it is based on a false belief. Nonetheless the response to placebo pain medication can sometimes be dramatic. In fact, the more intense the pain, the more effective placebos are (they do not work well in situations of minor pain): paradox in action. Moreover, placebos do not work very well if the person knows he or she is taking one. This is further paradox: success through ignorance.

In healing by prayer, paradox reigns supreme: There is no known explanation in mainstream science; the method is utterly unreasonable. This applies also to other distant phenomena we've looked at, including healing at a distance, EEG correlations between people, transpersonal imagery, and distant or intuitive diagnosis.

Paradox manifests most profoundly in so-called miracle cures. Again, there is no known mechanism for how they *can* occur, which is one of the reasons they are so frequently denied. Because of their sheer unreasonableness, miracles are a particular thorn in the flesh of current medical theories, all of which strive to be completely rational. But miracle cures keep happening in defiance of reason, as in the following example, which is one of the most recent cases to be certified as a miracle cure by the International Medical Committee of Lourdes.

Delizia Cirolli grew up on the slopes of Mount Etna in Sicily. In 1976, after her twelfth birthday, she noticed a painful swelling of her right knee and went to a physician. An X ray showed change in the bone, and she was referred to a well-known orthopedic specialist at the University of Catania. After further X rays a biopsy was taken, which showed that the lesion of the knee was a metastasis of a neuroblastoma, a highly malignant tumor. The surgeon advised amputation of the leg, but the family refused. He then advised cobalt irradiation, but Delizia was so unhappy her parents took her home the next day before any treatment was given. Other specialists were consulted, but no therapy was undertaken.

Delizia's teacher then suggested that she be taken to Lourdes, where a vision of the Virgin Mary appeared in 1858 to a fourteen-year-old girl, and where miraculous healings are purported to occur. Money was collected from other villagers to make the trip possible, and her mother took her to the shrine in August 1976. There she spent four days attending ceremonies, praying at the grotto, and bathing in the sacred waters. But there was no improvement, and by September X rays showed extension of the original tumor. Still, the villagers continued to pray for her cure, and her mother regularly gave her water from Lourdes.

Suddenly, before Christmas, Delizia announced she wanted to get up and go outside, which she proceeded to do without pain. But because of her weakness she did not get far, for by this time she weighed only forty-eight pounds. However, she continued gradually to improve. Her knee swelling eventually disappeared and her general condition returned to normal. X rays documented that the bone had repaired itself, and extensive studies revealed no other tumor throughout the body. The original biopsy was reviewed by French histologists eminent in the field of bone tumors. The final conclusion was that Delizia's tumor was not a neuroblastoma, as was originally suggested, but Ewing's tumor, another type of aggressive, malignant tumor affecting children. In either case, her response was remarkable: spontaneous remission of neuroblastoma has never been reported after the age of five, and spontaneous remission of Ewing's tumor has never been reported.[9]

Yet the paradoxical dimension in which miraculous, breakthrough healings occur is not *totally* paradoxical. There is usually *some* reasoning and doing involved. After all, Delizia made the journey to the shrine at Lourdes. But even so, active effort in the paradoxical domain is radically overshadowed by something that can never be described as "making it happen." At best, one can only set the stage. This means that we can never compel the universe to come to our terms but must, as the great psychologist C. G. Jung once said, wait patiently with gratitude and see what the universe wishes to give.

Being immersed in the paradoxical domain *feels* different. When we are swept up in paradox, the world seems changed. We are outside the usual causal and rational flow of events, and we know it. There may be a sense of oneness and unity, in which there is no "out there" that is being experienced but only "experience." During these moments, common-sense ideas such as the desirability of a long life and of the eradication of pain and death can undergo a transformation. Birth and death may be seen in new ways, losing their status as the absolute beginning and end of life—for "beginnings" and "endings" no longer make sense in the experience of the "eternal now." One senses that consciousness is more than the chaotic emotions and thoughts experienced at other moments; it feels still and quiet, independent of space and time and not a hostage of our ever-changing brain and body.

Ken Wilber, the transpersonal psychologist and philosopher, has described this experiential region as the domain of spirit. It has been elucidated by the mystics, visionaries, and seers of various religious traditions for millennia. As Wilber emphasizes, its language is *paradox*—which is simply what spirit looks like to the everyday mind. This domain contains the numinous feeling that one is nearing ultimates. And in it anything can happen. Even miracles.

But they don't *always* happen. If they did, they would hardly be paradoxical, and all we would have to do would be to follow some causal formula to bring them about. We seem always to be searching for this formula, some sure-fire way to set breakthrough healings in motion. But as already emphasized, in the domain of paradox where these particular healing events dwell, they are never fully predictable and they cannot be controlled.

SAINTS AND MYSTICS

Neither do miracles correlate with "being spiritual" as many people want to insist—which is further evidence of their paradoxical nature. A quick look at the lives of the spiritual geniuses—the saints and mystics—tells us this. If there were a one-to-one correlation between spiritual attainment and physical health, we might suspect that the saints and mystics would live long and healthy lives. Yet, not only do they die of the same diseases that afflict the rest of us (cancer, heart attacks, strokes, etc.), but frequently their lives are health disasters.

Three of the holiest men of this century have all died of cancer—the great teacher Krishnamurti (cancer of the pancreas); Ramana Maharshi, India's beloved saint (cancer of the stomach); and Suzuki Roshi, who helped bring Zen Buddhism to the United States and who established the San Francisco Zen Center (cancer of the stomach). Even Saint Bernadette, who in 1858 saw a vision of the Virgin Mary at Lourdes, did not herself experience a miraculous healing when she became sick. She died after grotesque suffering from bone cancer at the age of thirty-five.[10]

Although we do not know why great spiritual figures, such as the three great teachers mentioned above, die of the commonest problems, we can presume that it was not because they weren't "high" or "holy" enough, or because they did not meditate enough, or were not sufficiently God-realized. At some point in their spiritual path they seem to shift to a different calculus of health and illness, birth and death. As their statements and writings show, they do not view disease and death through the prism of tragedy as we do. They are at home in the domain of paradox, and thus able to comprehend that "the end" can be equally a beginning or a continuation. Here, then, is another paradox: miracles are not handed out freely to the "most spiritual."

The idea that one can "die whole" is an old theme in religious traditions. It is a mistake to think this happens only to "holy" people such as those just mentioned; common folk die whole as well. This has been an extraordinarily difficult lesson for me to learn as a physician. I have recoiled more than once on hearing someone say that "a healing took place" before the patient died. These comments always seemed to me desperate attempts of grieving families and friends to find solace by whatever means they could, including self-delusion. Associating healing and death appeared to me the ultimate in twisted logic. This reflected my own difficulty as a physician in learning to exist in paradox. In dealing with cases of life-threatening illness, I had learned to do, but not to be.

As usual in these matters, our patients are our teachers.

Molly was an elderly patient who had a host of medical problems along with an aversion to physicians. I got to know her in her final year. She had been enormously healthy most of her life and had raised three daughters. Now she was suffering from congestive heart failure and kidney failure but was on no medication. Following her first visit, I discussed her situation with her and one of her daughters.

"The good news is that there's a lot we can do," I assured her. "Why, you've never really been treated for any of this." I went on to describe her options: proper diet, medications, even dialysis if it came down to it. I expected her to react enthusiastically at the prospect of getting better, and was completely taken aback by her response.

"No thank you, Doctor," she said. "I don't want any of that."

"But Mom," her daughter interrupted, "it will make you feel better."

"I feel fine!" Molly rebutted. I wondered how this was possible; she had congestive heart failure and was continually short of breath.

"Mom, perhaps you're just depressed," her daughter offered. "We'll talk about it. Maybe some medication for depression. . . ."

But Molly would not budge. "Why do you insist I'm depressed and unhappy? Why do you think it's not O.K. to be sick? Or to die? You can't see through my eyes." At Molly's mention of her own death, her daughter burst into tears.

Through the weeks ahead Molly returned several times to my office, seemingly to appease her family members more than anything else. On each visit she seemed to be somewhere else. There was never a glimmer of disappointment, fear, or bitterness in anything she said or did. Molly, it seemed, was giving us a lesson.

Finally she was too sick to come to the office. Predictably, she refused to be hospitalized, wanting to die at home. I instructed her adoring daughters in how to procure a hospital bed and how to make her as comfortable as possible. They became superb home nurses.

The day Molly died, the daughter I'd met on Molly's first visit came to my office to let me know. She was tearful but content, knowing that she had carried out her mother's wishes to the letter.

"Mom wanted you to have this," she said, handing me a letter. "She managed to write it a couple of days ago."

I opened the envelope. In Molly's handwriting was a message such as I'd never received before. It said simply,

> Dear Dr. Dossey,
> Thank you for what you didn't do.
> Molly M.

It is easy enough to dismiss Molly's behavior as that of someone cantankerously at odds with the medical system. I think it goes deeper, however, and I think there may be a connection between Molly and the saints and mystics who seem also to be "somewhere else" in their attitudes to health. Earlier I said the saints and mystics had a different calculus of health and illness, a way of reckoning them that is foreign to most people. I believe Molly did also. But I do not mean that such people despise life and want to leave it. Indeed, some spiritual masters seem as reluctant as ordinary people to depart at death. The sociologist Kyriacos C. Markides, in his remarkable book *The Magus of Strovolos,* tells the story of a famous Zen master. He preached all his life about the unimportance and the illusory nature of the material world. When on his deathbed, his disciples gathered around him eager to hear some final words of wisdom. He said simply, "I want to live, I want to live." His followers were dismayed and protested, "But master, how can you say that?" "Really, really, I want to live," he repeated as he closed his eyes. Their master's final lesson: high spiritual attainment and "being human" are not incompatible.[11]

Another paradox in the way many spiritually aware people view health is that they believe illness and adversity are somehow *required* in our lives—as Emily Dickinson put it, "In insecurity to lie / Is joy's insuring quality." perhaps it was this understanding that led Matisse to say, "I have some right to defend my own pain. . . . I like to have an attack of pain now and then . . . —I could not explain it."[12] The Swiss psychologist C. G. Jung took a similar stand; he "could not imagine a fate more awful, a fate worse than death, than a life lived in perfect balance and harmony."[13] Matisse's and Jung's words are often misunderstood; they sound masochistic to many.

For Jung, the psyche is a continuous balancing act between the conscious and unconscious parts of ourselves. When one force gets the upper hand and crowds the other out, psychological disaster results. Jung maintained that the conscious, aware part of the psyche invariably prefers health and eschews illness, whereas the unconscious realizes that life is not so simple, that adversity—even illness—has its necessary place. If Jung is right, the question arises: Is "perfect health" desirable, since it totally excludes illness and adversity? Is it not a contradiction in terms?

The noted writer, explorer, and soldier, Sir Laurens van der Post, has written one of the best expositions of Jung's ideas. Van der Post suggested, along with Jung, that *anything* could be "too much of a good thing": "[Can we be] overgentle . . . ? . . . [Can] human beings be overgood and [is] goodness not subject also to the laws of proportion as all else and [must it not] be aware of its own excess?"[14] Similarly, anthropologist Gregory Bateson once said, "There is always an optimal value beyond which anything is toxic, *no matter what:* oxygen, sleep, psychotherapy, philosophy. Biological variables always need equilibrium [emphasis added]."[15]

The paradox, glimpsed occasionally by saints and mystics, psychologists and scientists, is that health and illness "go together," and even illness has its place. Although this may not be comforting to someone who is ill, it is not just overtheorizing but a truth embodied in the cells and molecules of our bodies. It is particularly evident in the human immune system. For a certain period following birth, we are protected from infections by the antibodies that originated in the body of our mother. But this "passive immunity" soon dwindles and we begin to develop our own resistance. This can be done only through repeated exposures to pathogens of various sorts—viruses, bacteria, fungi—that create temporary "mini-illnesses," which spur us to develop the appropriate immune responses. If this process does not take place, life is cut short by overwhelming infections. The paradox, carved into our biology: life and health depend on illness and cannot exist without it.

In the lives of many persons such as Molly above, this paradoxical realization becomes fully conscious. When it does, it is *never* just an intellectual understanding. Those who experience it describe it as a source of great peace, certainty, and clarity. Almost invariably it is accompanied by deeper understandings not just about illness but about the nature of death itself—death as transformation, as a bridge between two dimensions of human experience.

IS EMPTINESS REALLY EMPTY?

We have repeatedly noted that the psychological state that seems to set the stage for breakthrough healings is that of emptiness, a kind of psychological void, a mode of being where acceptance, attunement, and alignment eclipse all forms of doing. Some people strenuously object to this psychological state. I was once invited to discuss the concept on a radio talk show. As illustrations of how this "void" could be helpful physically, I described the healthful changes that can come about through meditation and biofeedback, both of which promote it. I was assailed by several callers, all making the same point: when we let our guard down, nothing good can happen. Psychological emptiness is an open door and entry point to "the devil," and it can only lead to harm.

This point of view is by no means confined to Christian fundamentalists. It seems a characteristic of the Western mind to mistrust the void. We equate it with dissolution, extermination, and death. It conjures images of an unending, black nothingness, and evokes fear and loathing in us.

Other cultures have an entirely different understanding of the void. Among these are the native tribes of the Pacific Northwest. Some of these tribes carve gigantic, elaborate totem poles with large holes in the center. Springing from and encircling the holes are major life forms including human infants. The void is seen as the *plenum,* the fecund source of all life.

Dr. Renée Weber, philosopher and professor at Rutgers University, has applied a similar concept to the domain of healing. In her seminal paper "Philosophical Foundations and Frameworks for Healing," she has proposed that there is an implicit ordering principle at the foundation of existence—a certain wholeness and perfection that surfaces under propitious conditions. The role of the healer is to facilitate this process—to call forth the right order from the void. Weber traces the tradition of an inherent wholeness or perfection in the world from the sixty century B.C., beginning with the Sankhya philosophy of ancient India, through the yoga system of Patanjali, through Buddhism, and into the Western models set forth by Plato, Pythagoras, and Spinoza. Seen against the backdrop of these historical traditions, our notion of the void as nothingness and death may seem like a historical aberration.[16]

THERAPIES OF BEING

One of the most tantalizing bits of evidence that different ways of being can catalyze profound changes in one's body comes from persons with multiple personality syndrome, discussed earlier ("The Siege of Shame: Multiple Personality Disorder"). In these cases, the *genetics* of the person doesn't change from personality to personality; he or she still has the same body. What does change is the sense of *being*—and along with it, allergies, pain, immune function, handedness, menstrual cycles, cerebral dominance, facility for foreign languages, and even diabetes. Currently the connection between multiples' "shifts of being" and changes in their body, particularly the immune system, is the subject of research at various institutions.[17] Could these scientific studies lead someday to "therapies of being" instead of therapies of doing? Could they shed light on the mechanisms underlying miracles, spontaneous remissions, and placebo responses? Instead of prescribing medication, surgery, and radiation, might physicians someday prescribe "changes in being" as confidently as they now prescribe physical interventions? Could "existential therapy" someday take its place alongside internal medicine and surgery as an appropriate form of treatment for even the most serious diseases? These directions are clearly implied by the strange paradoxical healings that litter the annals of our best medical literature, and the cases that crop up from time to time in every physician's experience.

Hippocrates said: "What you should put first in all the practice of your art is how to make the patient well; and if he can be made well in many ways, one should choose the least troublesome."

Many health problems such as broken bones, traumatic amputations, and life-threatening infections call overwhelmingly for "doing therapies," which we would be foolish to abandon without good alternatives. But sometimes the "least troublesome" treatments are the "being therapies." If they ever become accepted, we may wonder why we preferred the troublesome "doing therapies" for so long. And if we are to honor "being therapies," a fundamental change in our *own* being must occur—a willingness to stand in paradox instead of rationality, and a willingness to be, yes, *wrong*. A famous modern physician, William B. Bean, once expressed this requirement: "The one mark of maturity, especially in a physician, and perhaps it is even rarer in a scientist, is the capacity to deal with uncertainty." The domain of paradoxical healing *is* uncertain. It does not follow the predictable, deterministic patterns we physicians have learned to prefer in our treatment algorithms. But if some of the certainty and control are lost in the shift toward "being therapies," something more is gained in the bargain: the wondrous, the glorious, the *miraculous*.

By any measure, a good trade.

The Secret Helper:
The Invisible Power Within

[I have] a growing . . . sense of some entirely lively entity within, an entity unchanged from milk-and-crackers in the first grade through lumberjacking, Popsicle packing, book publishing, news reporting, sexual encounters, spiritual exercises, loving and angry relations, laughter until the tears came and vice versa, and on and on until right this minute. . . . For me, this "entity" is not wishful thinking, but it is impossible to name. My experience is that it is incapable of piety or misdeed, intellectual or emotional acrobatics, yet it informs all things.

—ADAM FISHER[1]

Walter Dent was ninety-seven years old, for many years the oldest patient in my practice. He was an enigma, one of the most inscrutable patients I have ever known.

Walt was crippled with arthritis in both knees, and he ambulated with a cane in each hand. Although they would have simplified his difficulties, crutches were to him an anathema and a wheelchair unthinkable. In spite of his considerable problems it usually was unclear to me why he came to the office for periodic visits: he declared my physical examinations a waste of time, declined all lab tests, despised medication, and refused to take anything I prescribed.

"Walt, why do you come to see me?" I asked him one day. "You never do anything I say."

"Because you're a nice boy," he responded with a smile. "You might learn something."

When he hobbled into the office on another occasion, I asked him if he finally had decided to take the arthritis medication I once again was attempting to prescribe.

"Of course not!" he said. "Why should I? I'm ninety-seven years old. You have to admit that *something*'s working. And it's not your pills."

Walt had immense personal charm which he unfailingly lavished on the office nursing staff, who responded in kind. On each visit he would inquire about their children, spouses, and love affairs with sincere interest and concern. He always remembered these details from visit to visit. In effect, Walt was functioning as a counselor. This was ironic: the crippled patient taking care of the healthy professionals. Because these "therapy sessions" seemed endless and always derailed the office schedule, I learned to schedule Walt as the last patient of the day.

Walt had an unerring sense of an inner healing strength. It was the "something" that was stronger than my pills, the power that had helped him come this far. Although he could not explicitly discuss it, on occasion he would allude to this interior force when one of the nurses invariably would ask him "the secret" to his longevity.

"Yes, there is a secret. But if I told you, it wouldn't be a secret, would it?" Walt relished the question and his mischievous reply never varied.

He soon got the chance to put his "secret" to work. Shortly before his hundredth birthday, he fell one wintry day and broke his hip. I called an orthopedic surgeon to take care of the problem. While in the emergency room Walt proved to be his usual enigmatic self. Soon the orthopedist, who had not previously met him, was on the phone. He was obviously agitated.

"This guy's got to be in a lot of pain, but I can't get him to take anything for it. Says he has a 'secret' he prefers to use. Think you can come down and reason with him?" Walt was being Walt.

I arrived in the emergency room as Walt was being prepared for surgery. In marked contrast to his irritated surgeon, he was completely placid, as if nothing unusual were happening.

"I hear you're still using your secret, Walt."

"Why not? It's worked for almost a hundred years," he said. "Look, Doc, I'm going away for a few days. See you when I get back. In the meantime, you tell this young surgeon, 'no pills and no shots.'" Walt then closed his eyes.

"Walt, what the hell are you talking about?" I demanded, but could elicit no response. Walt was somewhere else. Our conversation obviously was over.

For four days following surgery Walt slept in perfect repose without the benefit of any "pills or shots" for pain. His recovery was flawless, with no complications. On the fifth day I stopped by his room. He was awake and alert.

"Welcome back," I said. "By the way, Walt, where did you go?" As soon as he heard my words, I saw a twinkle in his eyes and I knew what was coming.

"If I told you, it wouldn't be a secret, would it?"

While I was there, the nurses from my office came by to pay Walt a group visit. Their affection for the arthritic old man was touching. Surrounding him on either side, they adoringly chattered, stroked his forehead, fluffed his pillow, and inspected his surgical site. But before long Walt, as usual, took control of the conversation and began interrogating them about the personal concerns they had shared with him in his latest office "therapy session." After a half-hour their visit ended.

Walt continued to recover uneventfully and lived for several more years. His reliance on his intrinsic healing capacity never wavered. I continued to badger him to elaborate on his secret, but he steadfastly refused any discussion. I am not sure he could have verbalized about it even if he had wished. It did not matter: Walt's inner invisible helper did not require being dressed in language for its power.

One of the most significant possible breakthroughs in understanding how healing comes about is the realization that we all possess an inner source of healing and strength that operates behind the scenes with no help whatsoever from our conscious mind. This "secret helper" has not been given its due. The bulk of advice given today under the rubric of "self-help" implies that the conscious, aware part of ourselves is responsible for healing us. Our entire culture is mesmerized by the belief that only by hard work and *conscious* effort can we accomplish what we desire. Conscious effort *is* important. But beyond our awareness is a superb back-up system that comes "factory installed," on "automatic," ready to help at any time.

Writer Aldous Huxley discovered this behind-the-scenes power in his own life, and called it his "not-I." He described it thus:

> Total awareness . . . reveals the following facts: that I am profoundly ignorant, that I am impotent to the point of helplessness and that the most valuable elements in my personality are unknown qualities existing "out there," as mental objects more or less completely independent of my control. This discovery may seem at first rather humiliating and even depressing. But if I wholeheartedly accept them, the facts become a source of peace, a reason for serenity and cheerfulness. I am ignorant and impotent and yet, somehow or other, here I am, but alive and kicking. In spite of everything, I survive, I get by, sometimes I even get on. From those two sets of facts—my survival on the one hand and my ignorance and impotence on the other—I can only infer that the not-I, which looks after my body and gives me my best ideas, must be amazingly intelligent, knowledgeable and strong. As a self-centered ego, I do my best to interfere with the beneficent workings of this not-I. But in spite of my likes and dislikes, in spite of my malice, my infatuations, my gnawing anxieties . . . this not-I, with whom I am associated, sustains me, preserves me, gives me a long succession of second chances. We know very little and can achieve very little; but we are at liberty, if we so choose, to co-operate with a greater power and a completer knowledge, an unknown quantity at once immanent and transcendent, at once physical and mental, at once subjective and objective. If we co-operate we shall be all right, even if the worst should happen. If we refuse to cooperate, we shall be all wrong even in the most propitious circumstances.[2]

To a generation being told it has consciously to pull itself up by its own bootstraps, Huxley's observations may be empowering. This not-I, of which I am unaware, can be a more potent helper than my conscious I. Even better, it is apparently benevolent most of the time. Rather than being in tight-fisted control at all times, I only have to cooperate. Realizing this, the pressure eases and I can relax. As I become more friendly with this part of myself, I gradually develop a tolerance for paradox; I realize the truth in the observation of psychologist Patricia Sun that, "The more conscious you become, the more unconscious you realize you are."

How does this secret helper manifest itself in health and illness? We've already seen it surface many times. In the case of the "fishskin boy" whose congenital disease responded to hypnosis, it was the unconscious, unaware part of the mind that mediated his astonishing improvement. In the cases of psychic healing, some inner superintelligence was set in motion that somehow bypassed intellectual, rational understanding. This secret helper was particularly obvious in those cases in which completely unconscious, anesthetized patients were given suggestions that later improved their health. In *none* of these instances is the conscious I in control of what is happening. *Whatever* is happening—and there are great unknowns in this process—the bulk of the action lies almost totally outside conscious awareness.

The secret helper is so intent on preserving us it seems it will stop at nothing. It is not constrained by the rules of conduct and propriety that govern our *conscious* conduct. One of its favorite and most effective devices is creating a lie that surfaces eventually in our awareness. When it does so, the lie is often called *denial*. Denial is a blatant rejection of the way things are, a repudiation of reality. As offensive as this may be to many, it is becoming abundantly clear that denial can save lives.

Nowhere is the value of denial more apparent than in the coronary care unit following heart attack, where it has been shown that the *higher* the denial, the *lower* the mortality.[3] Persons who deny being frightened, who minimize the seriousness of their illness, and who give the appearance of generally being unruffled tend to survive the CCU experience in larger numbers than those who are appropriately worried or who are unable to deny their distress. These findings led Dr. Thomas P. Hackett of Harvard Medical School, a pioneer in this research, to observe that "While denial can play the role of the enemy to the myocardial infarction victim in delaying his arrival in the emergency ward, it can also serve as an ally in the CCU."[4]

As Hacket implies, there are obviously times in which denial can be deadly, as when a person with chest pain says, "It's just indigestion," or "This can't be a heart attack; I'm too young for that to happen," and delays seeking medical care. Indeed, denial is one of the reasons why 50 percent of people with heart attacks die before reaching the hospital. But once inside the hospital it's another matter. Here denial lowers psychological and physiological tension. It reduces the levels of adrenaline in the blood and lowers the sensitivity of the injured heart to the development of potentially fatal irregularities of its rhythm.

If denial is consciously chosen, however, it ceases to be genuine—for we cannot consciously fool ourselves into *not* believing something exists, once the believe is already lodged in consciousness. Thus it is useless for the heart attack victim who finds himself in the coronary care unit to say to himself, "Statistics show that if I deny my heart attack, I'll have a better chance of surviving. So I'm going to close my eyes, lie back, and start denying!" It's like trying to not think of a pink elephant: we're defeated before we start. In a sense, instead of our choosing denial, denial must choose us. This implies that the secret helper makes its own rules; we cannot compel it or tell it what to do.

An internal, unconscious dishonesty can be a valuable psychological strategy for some persons with cancer as well.

Researcher Keith W. Pettingale and his colleagues at King's College School of Medicine and Dentistry in London studied the psychological response of women three months after mastectomy. At a five-year follow-up, they found that the rate of recurrence-free survival was significantly higher among patients who had reacted to their cancer either with a fighting spirit or with denial than among those who had reacted with stoic acceptance or feelings of hopelessness and helplessness. There was no evidence that this finding was due to initial biological differences, since these patient groups were similar in terms of clinical stage, the size of the tumor, its cancerous grade, its appearance on mammograms, and their hormonal and immunological profiles. After a followup period of ten years, the outcome was the same: those patients

demonstrating a fighting spirit or denial did better and had higher rates
of survival.[5]

When life is running smoothly we may feel that denial is a reprehen-
sible psychological tactic, a tactic that only those lacking the courage
to "face reality" would employ. But psychologist Shelley E. Taylor
of UCLA has discovered that almost anyone will adopt a coping
strategy based in illusion if life becomes difficult enough. As a result
of her work with cancer and cardiac patients, rape victims, and other
individuals facing life-threatening happenings, Taylor suggests that
the readjustment process following crisis focuses around three
themes: a search for meaning in the experience, an attempt to regain
mastery over the event in particular and over one's life more
generally, and an effort to enhance one's self-esteem—to feel good
about oneself again in spite of the personal setback. The ability to
accomplish these goals, Taylor states, is not rare; in fact it is a
"formidable" resource possessed by most persons and constitutes one
of the most impressive qualities of the human psyche. Even after
enormous problems such as personal illness or the death of a loved
one, the majority of people achieve a quality of life or level of
happiness equivalent to or even greater than their prior level. Most
adjust largely on their own; typically, they do not seek professional
help but use their social networks and individual resources.

One of the most effective strategies used to find meaning, regain
mastery, and restore self-esteem following tragedy is what Taylor
calls "illusion." By "illusion" Taylor does not mean that one believes
a lie, but that one may look at the facts in a particular light, choosing
a slant that yields a positive picture instead of a negative one. For
instance, over half of Taylor's cancer patients reported that the cancer
experience was a good thing because it had caused them to reappraise
their lives. For many, this meant a new attitude to life that was more
fulfilling and worthwhile. Many of the patients developed theories
about why they got cancer that may or may not have had a basis in
fact—for example, attributing their cancer to diet or to some medication they had taken. By positing such a cause, they could reinstate
a sense of self-mastery by changing their diet or eliminating the feared
medication.

Another strategy used by most cancer patients, Taylor found, is to make *selective comparisons* with other persons with the same disease. Women with breast cancer tended to compare themselves with other women with cancer who were doing poorly, which enhanced their estimation of their own strengths. This "downward comparison" was so important that if a proper "comparison target" was not present, these women would manufacture a norm according to which other women were worse off than they were.

Summing up, Taylor states, "The effective individual in the face of threat . . . seems to be one who permits the development of illusions, nurtures those illusions, and is ultimately restored by those illusions." But if illusions *are* restorative and if denial *is* lifesaving, as the evidence shows, why do we object so strenuously to their use? As Taylor notes, those who hold them are said to be weak-willed or ignorant, and are frequently portrayed in literature as self-deluded, naive, or pathetic creatures. (Relevant literary examples are found in works ranging from Cervantes's *Don Quixote,* O'Neill's *The Iceman Cometh* and Albee's *Who's Afraid of Virginia Woolf.*) Taylor maintains we need a different attitude: "Illusions can have a dynamic force. They can simultaneously protect and prompt constructive thought and action. . . . Normal cognitive processing and behavior may depend on a substantial degree of illusion, whereas the ability to see things clearly can be associated with depression and inactivity. Thus, far from impeding adjustment, illusion may be essential for adequate coping."[6]

Another device used by the secret helper is excuses. Excuses, like denial, are an evasion of reality. Evidence suggests that they, too, can serve a valuable function. Research by psychologists C. R. Snyder and Raymond Higgins at the University of Kansas has shown that persons who offer themselves plausible excuses have greater self-esteem, better health, and perform better on all sorts of cognitive, social, and physical tasks than people who put the blame on themselves when things go wrong. Snyder and Higgins believe that excuses are a distancing process, a way of placing the blame for failure on external factors rather than on our own lack of competence or intelligence. While excuses don't eradicate our sense of failure completely, they nonetheless make our failures less troubling. They help preserve a sense of self-worth and personal integrity—as when we say that we flunked a test because we didn't study hard enough, not because we weren't intelligent enough. Excuse makers not only don't blame themselves, they also tend to view their setbacks as temporary. Excuses give them time to marshal additional psychological resources for the next challenge. Audiences even collaborate with excuse makers by endorsing their phony version of reality, as if there is some collective attempt to preserve the person's threatened sense of worth. Snyder and Higgins conclude that excuses are far from the "simple, silly and ineffective ploys" most people consider them to be and are, in fact, necessary illusions.[7]

This is not to extol denial, excuses, and dishonesty in dealing with illness. In fact, as a physician I am not attracted to these ways of structuring one's reality and I, like most other people, would like to believe that honesty will always work better than sticking one's head in the sand. But the facts say otherwise, and to imply that honesty always works best is simply untrue. It appears that sometimes our potent, unconscious "assist device" does not care a whit about our preferred versions of reality—whether we employ honesty, openness, or downright denial and illusion.

Many persons believe the above studies reveal the world's perversity, in that self-deceit and dishonesty are rewarded, but this view seems the height of ingratitude. The opposite may be true: the universe in fact may be showing us its benevolence by saying, "I give you not one but *many* ways to survive difficult situations—some conscious, some unconscious. Pick the method that suits you best; if you fail, I stand ready to help."

Today in many "holisitic" health care circles an enormous emphasis is placed on the idea that "you create your own reality." The intent is noble, that of creating a sense of responsibility for one's health. However, the questions that almost never get asked by the advocates of this idea are, "What do you mean by 'you'? Who is this 'self' that creates?" Invariably it is the conscious I that is being referred to, which can never be in complete control even if it desires.

I have presented to many holistic health meetings the studies showing that strategies of denial and illusion *work*. People are generally disturbed by these findings. I understand this response; *I*, too, am troubled by them. But the data will not go away in deference to our egos, and we must try to learn the lessons being offered.

Patricia Sun underscores the problem inherent in emphasizing total self-responsibility, and speaks for a broader view:

> The thing . . . now is to talk about how "you created it." It gets a little annoying [because] there's something missing there . . . you are an effect of this universe and . . . you are completely in response to it, receptive to it.
>
> As you paradoxically let yourself be empty and say, "I don't know," you make a wonderful space to be filled, and as you are filled you expand and you are greater. . . . You win by simultaneously knowing you are a pipsqueak in the universe, you don't know anything. . . . The minute you realize the paradox inherent in our perception of the universe, you will have broadened your ability to perceive the universe.[8]

As long as we tell ourselves that we are the creators of our entire reality and that we are completely responsible for anything that happens, we set ourselves up for a sense of guilt, shame, and failure when things don't work out as we planned, as Carol's case showed earlier (pages 29–30). What is perhaps worse, as long as our energy is expended in endlessly trying to shape and control every aspect of our destiny, we are likely to miss subtle messages from the world, including from our own unconscious. There is another way—a way that honors the mysteries of the unconscious self and its connection to the world. Perceiving this connection requires a degree of letting go and relinquishing conscious control. It entails trust and acceptance, attunement and alignment, with "what is." One of the clearest expressions in modern literature of this state of awareness and the joy that comes is in Hermann Hesse's *Siddhartha,* when Siddhartha learns to see the world in a new way:

> Siddhartha listened. He was now listening intently, completely absorbed, quite empty, taking in everything. He felt that he had now completely learned the art of listening. He had often heard all this before, all these numerous voices in the river, but today they sounded different. He could no longer distinguish the different voices—the merry voice from

the weeping voice, the childish voice from the manly voice. They all belonged to each other: the lament of those who yearn, the laughter of the wise, the cry of indignation and groan of the dying. They were all interwoven and interlocked, entwined in a thousand ways. And all the voices, all the goals, all the yearnings, all the sorrows, all the pleasures, all the good and evil, all of them together was the world. All of them together was the stream of events, the music of life. When Siddhartha listened attentively to the river, to this song of a thousand voices: when he did not listen to the sorrow or laughter, when he did not blind his soul to any one particular voice and absorb it in his Self, but heard them all, the whole, the unity; then the great song of a thousand voices consisted of one word: Om—perfection.[9]

Do secret helpers exist beyond the unconscious mind? One person who thought so was Nobel physicist Erwin Schrödinger, whose wave equations lie at the heart of modern physics. Schrödinger believed in a secret helper who was powerful enough to ensure *immortality*. This secret helper is not part of the unconscious mind; it is the earth itself:

Thus you can throw yourself flat on the ground, stretched out on Mother Earth, with the certain conviction that you are one with her and she with you. You are as firmly established, as invulnerable as she, indeed a thousand times more invulnerable. As surely as she will engulf you tomorrow, so surely will she bring you forth anew to new striving and suffering. And not merely "some day": now, today, every day she is bringing you forth, not *once* but thousands of times, just as every day she engulfs you a thousand times over. For eternally and always there is only *now*, one and the same now; the present is the only thing that has no end.[10]

TWENTY-ONE

The Hospital Experience:
How to Be a Survivor

As a physician I have a natural antipathy for the dozens of books that engage in reckless, irresponsible doctor- and hospital-bashing. Most are sensationalistic and only thinly disguise the author's anger. But as someone who has spent most of his life caring for patients in hospitals, I realize that some of these books contain more than a grain of truth. Hospitals *are* dangerous places. Sick people die in them, but perfectly healthy people do, too. And it is astonishing how *little* it takes to kill an individual. Sometimes a word will do.

A fifty-one-year-old schoolteacher, recently retired, underwent a radical neck operation for cancer, in which her voice box and most of the neck muscles were removed. She did well afterward. In only two weeks she had learned to suction her own secretions, feed herself by tube, and change her own dressings. She was making plans to move to a new home with her husband and enroll in a special class to learn esophageal speech. The evening before her expected discharge, her surgeon came by as usual. In trying to help her face the future realistically, he told her that although all the tumor in the neck had been removed, other tumors existed elsewhere that could not be excised. Her life expectancy, he said, was nine to twelve months. After the well-intentioned surgeon left, the woman slumped into her chair, refused to eat or suction herself, and said simply, "I want to go to bed." Three days later she died.[1]

Sometimes it is not what is said or done by others but the emotions and fears we bring to the hospital experience that are destructive, as in the following case.

> A twenty-five-year-old man who was about to be married was admitted to the hospital for a routine circumcision. He received the usual preoperative chest X ray, electrocardiogram, blood work, and physical examination and was pronounced to be "in perfect health." The night before surgery his nurse heard him say, "I'm scared to death." Although the remark did not mean anything to her when it was made, it was burned into her memory when, during surgery the next day, he experienced a cardiac arrest and died on the table.[2]

For some people, the thought of becoming a hospital patient is among the most terrifying imaginable. Fear of hospitals is not rare; everyone feels it to some degree. When the fear is strong, learning ways to deal with it can be an enormous—even lifesaving—breakthrough.

People are beginning to discover steps they can take to survive the hospital experience. They are rejecting the belief that hospitals are unchangeable, monolithic structures completely outside their influence. They see themselves as consumers with the power to hire and fire and dictate many of their own terms.

Some hospitals *are* "different." Some have found creative ways to annul the fear and apprehension that patients feel on entering them. Perhaps the most famous is Planetree, a thirteen-bed medical-surgical unit in San Francisco's Pacific Presbyterian Medical Center (Hippocrates taught his followers the art of medicine under a sycamore or planetree). Planetree is setting a new standard for patient-oriented care. It was started in 1985 by Angelica Thieriot following her own painful experiences as a hospital patient. The staff is painstaking in its attempts to dispel the mystery surrounding a patient's experience. Patients can request a survey of the pertinent medical literature from the Planetree library, giving them a chance to "read up" on their illness. Nurses are available to interpret anything that might not be clear. The nursing staff is highly selected; only nurses committed to the Planetree philosophy work on the unit. Planetree *looks* different: colors, lighting, carpeting, furniture, fabrics, and the absence of sharp corners create a warm, nurturing environment. Intrusive, jarring hospital items are hidden away—including bandage carts, chart racks, linen carts, and medical technological equipment. The nurses' station is in full view of the patients and is continually open to them; nurses and physicians are not sequestered behind walls of any sort. Visiting hours at Planetree are whenever the *patient* wants visitors. A patient lounge and comfortable surroundings encourage family and visitors to stay near. Relatives and friends who can do so are taught to participate in patient care before and after hospitalization. Patients can cook for themselves in the unit's kitchen, and a nutritionist assists them if they want advice on the best foods for their recovery. There is a piano and an art program, and patients may choose pictures for their walls from an "art cart." Another unique aspect of the unit is that patients can read their medical charts and may add their own observations, responses, and feelings. Not all doctors are allowed to admit patients and work on the Planetree unit; like the nurses, they must subscribe to the Planetree philosophy. Recognizing that the mind is a potent factor in getting well, and that attitudes and feelings make a difference, Planetree provides a special "high-touch" feature for patients: seven massage therapists are available in addition to the nursing staff.

Does it sound too good to be true? Planetree is indeed a breakthrough in hospital philosophy and design. It has achieved national prominence among hospital administrators and designers, in part because of its enormous popularity. Today hospitals vie with each other for "customers." Anything that "sells" attracts attention. Here is what a Planetree patient had to say:

> I cannot begin to express my appreciation for this wonderful unit. I really don't feel like I'm in a hospital . . . with all the funny smells, and nurses two halls away. The people here have been wonderful and I'm getting better care than I ever imagined. I really feel like I have a say in my own healing process. I hope this idea spreads to other hospitals.[3]

Spread it has. The director of Planetree, Ms. Robin Orr, is an active consultant to interested hospitals all over North America and Europe, and many hospitals are already in the process of adopting the Planetree model.

Still, most hospitals haven't come up to the Planetree standard. If yours is one of them and you're headed to the hospital, what are your options?

The first step is to realize that all hospitals are businesses, whether they acknowledge it or not. This means they are concerned with attracting "customers" and satisfying them. Although you may not have realized it, you have clout.

With a little effort and ingenuity you can plan your hospital stay in ways that can increase your peace of mind as well as your chances of doing well while there. Here are some things to consider.

Medical Surroundings

Be concerned what your room will look like. Insist on being told by the admissions clerk which room you will occupy, and if possible, visit it before checking into the hospital.

The pictures on the wall *do* make a difference! My most vivid lesson in this regard came during my internship, the year of intensive training that follows completion of medical school. In many hospitals the intern's hours are unbelievably long, the "on-call" responsibility lasting up to forty-eight sleepless hours without a break. During this time the intern cares for a ward full of sick persons, admits an unending stream of new patients, and fields life-or-death emergencies. But interns are a hardy lot, and they find ingenious ways to survive the ordeal. One of the most common coping strategies is "gallows" humor, which involves seeing the absurd or humorous side of even the most gruesome, hopeless situations.

A typical example occurred when I was assigned to the coronary care unit. America's space program was in full swing at the time, and the hospital's feeble attempts at decor reflected this fact. Hanging on a wall of Room 3 was a poster-size picture of a gigantic rocket blasting off from NASA's launching pad, flames and smoke billowing from its base. I do not profess to understand the inner workings of the minds of hospital designers, but I presume this picture was selected to provide visual distraction and a positive psychological stimulus— perhaps to convey a sense of control, hope, or power to the patient who, like the rocket, was loaded down in abundance with sophisticated electronic gadgets.

It didn't work. Room 3 became notorious for having more than its share of cardiac arrests. These became so routine that the macabre humor of the interns finally took over. In perfect harmony with the spirit of the picture, if patient Smith was doing poorly, his "countdown" had begun. An actual cardiac arrest became a "blast-off." If all attempts to resuscitate Smith failed, the "mission" was paradoxically judged to be successful, as Smith had "blasted off" and was now "in orbit." If, on the other hand, the resuscitation was successful and Smith survived, "blast-off [was] canceled, the mission aborted, and the launch rescheduled."

Did the rocket picture have something to do with the curse that seemed to afflict Room 3? My fellow interns and I had been taught that heart attacks, arrhythmias, and cardiac arrests were due entirely to physical factors, so we let the picture remain. The heart did not have eyes, and pictures, whether on the wall or in the mind, could have nothing to do with concrete, physical events.

I began to wonder what would happen if this violent scene were replaced with a picture of a pastoral setting, a high mountain lake, or a waterfall. Would the incidence of cardiac arrests diminish? Unknown to me at the time, other people were also thinking about whether the view from a hospital bed affects healing. I was astonished to learn, after all those countdowns and blast-offs in Room 3, that someone had actually done a scientific experiment to investigate this question. And the investigator was not a doctor but a *geographer,* Roger S. Ulrich, of the University of Delaware.

Ulrich examined the records of forty-six patients who underwent cholecystectomy (surgical removal of the gallbladder) in a suburban Pennsylvania hospital between 1972 and 1981. The patients were divided into two groups: half were in rooms from which they could look out on a small stand of deciduous trees, and the other half in rooms from which only a brown brick wall was visible. In all other respects the groups were comparable—the same nurses cared for both groups, and they were matched according to sex, age, smoking, obesity, and general level of previous health. All the cases examined were surgeries done between May 1 and October 20, the period during which the trees had foliage.

The trees appeared to make a major difference. Those patients with a view of them had shorter postoperative hospital stays, had fewer negative evaluations by their nurses, took fewer painkillers, and had lower scores for minor postsurgical complications.

Ulrich acknowledged that trees may not mean the same thing to everyone and that for some persons a lively city street might be more stimulating and therapeutic. This study does *not* mean, therefore, that all hospital rooms should be the same, or that all hospitals should have trees planted outside windows. It does mean, though, that the simplest, most ordinary perceptions have a way of entering the body and influencing rates of healing and degrees of pain.

Most persons would never think of having an operation without first checking out the surgeon. But what about the view from the room or the pictures on the wall? If the design and decor of hospital rooms affect the postoperative course, why should patients tolerate random room assignments? Why should hospitals *want* to assign rooms randomly? Since they currently can be penalized financially for longer hospital stays, why shouldn't they capitalize on the fact that pleasant views can facilitate earlier discharge and minimize complications? Why should pictures in rooms be fixed? Why not rotate them according to the patient's choice? It should be no more expensive to change a picture on a wall than to change the sheets on the bed, and the pictures never need laundering.[4]

Getting It Out

There are a variety of ways in which new meanings can be introduced into the medical experience—whether of having tests or a physical examination, having surgery, or undergoing anesthesia. The most important initial step in bringing new meaning to the medical experience is to admit that apprehension or fear exists, and to discuss it openly with the physician. Sometimes just getting one's worries onto the table is all that is required to alleviate them.

Music

Music can be a great solace in the modern hospital. Dr. Cathie Guzzetta, chairperson of the Department of Cardiovascular Nursing at Catholic University of America in Washington, D.C., has shown that listening to a music cassette tape can reduce the incidence of cardiac complications in patients in the coronary care unit.[5] Being admitted to a coronary care unit with a presumptive diagnosis of an acute myocardial infarction is an enormously stressful experience. If music can calm the mind and body in this situation, it can work in almost any setting.

Music preference is an important issue. What one person considers soothing may be unpleasant and annoying to another. Guzzetta allowed patients to choose between three types of music: soothing classical music, soothing popular music, and nontraditional music (compositions having no vocalization or meter, periods of silence, and an asymmetric rhythm). They listened to the music via headsets with a battery powered portable "Walkman"-type stereo recorder. Significant results were seen in only three twenty-minute listening sessions over a two-day period.

This approach is applicable to almost any medical experience in which the person is conscious. It is highly unobtrusive and makes no demands on the professional staff, because the music is channeled only to the patient. Because of music's universal appeal, most professionals intuitively understand its value and do not object to its use.

In the hospital, one can be one's own music therapist. Portable headsets are inexpensive and unobtrusive, and permit music selection on an individual basis.

Behavioral Anesthesia

The greatest fear for many hospitalized persons is the period during which they are under anesthesia. Here loss of control is complete. They may be suspended helplessly between life and death, their fate entirely in the hands of someone else. What can one do to diminish these apprehensions?

Many surgeons and anesthesiologists have recognized that a person undergoing general anesthesia can be adversely affected by their comments. Offhand, careless, or negative words apparently can become embedded in the subconscious mind of the anesthetized person and impede recovery, even though they are not consciously remembered on awakening. On the other hand, some persons seem highly susceptible to *positive* comments during this unconscious period. Awareness of these effects has led an increasing number of patients to ask their surgeons to exercise care about what is said during the operation. Others go further and ask their surgeons to give them positive suggestions while they are anesthetized. For example, the surgeon might say: "You will awake with little pain"; "Your healing will be complete"; "You will have a perfect surgical result"; "You will never experience this problem again"; or "You'll be back to work in six weeks."

Dr. Henry Bennett, of the Department of Anesthesiology at the University of California School of Medicine at Davis, describes a woman who requested that her hand be held during her anesthesia and that she be given words of encouragement, relaxation, and calm. Things were going well during the earlier stage of anesthesia, but suddenly she began vomiting when the surgeon, whom she consciously liked and respected, entered the room. He exited to scrub, and she quieted down, only to resume vomiting when he entered the room again. At this point the anesthesiologist suggested that the surgeon refrain from the loud argumentative behavior he was engaging in, as any evidence of psychological conflict might induce further vomiting or an even more serious stress response. "The surgeon behaved himself like a gentleman at a dinner party," Dr. Bennett relates. "His patient did well and made such quick progress that he requested in writing that this type of service [hand holding, relaxing and encouraging words, and decorous behavior] . . . be given to all his patients."[6]

These developments are encompassed in what has become known as "behavioral anesthesia." In addition to the precise use of drugs and anesthetic gases, anesthesiologists knowledgeable in this area strive for the precise use of *psychological* agents—communication signals, gestures, nonverbal posturing, touching, music, and verbal comments and suggestions. These begin with the first preoperative visit and extend through the administration of anesthesia, the surgery itself, the patient's emergence from anesthesia, and the period of recovery.[7]

The sheer simplicity of these measures is striking. For example, in one study, simple gestures meant to convey love and caring made a significant difference in the experience of surgery: women surgical patients whose hand was held by a nurse while their blood pressure and temperature were taken actually left the hospital sooner and recovered faster at home.[8]

An experiment showing how the meaning of surgery for the patient can be changed through simple means was done by anesthesiologist Lawrence D. Egbert and his colleagues at Massachusetts General Hospital.[9] The study involved ninety-seven patients who were to undergo some type of abdominal surgery (e.g., a gallbladder operation or stomach surgery). One group of forty-six patients was visited by the anesthesiologist before surgery and was clearly told what they could expect in the postoperative period. The physicians were explicit and honest about the pain that would occur, and taught them how to relax, how to take deep breaths, and how to move around in bed so they would remain more comfortable. They explained that the pain was caused by spasm in the abdominal muscles under the incision, and that they could control to a large extent the amount of spasm that would occur. Then the patients were revisited during the afternoon following the operation and again on the next two days, during which the information was reinforced.

The hospital course of this group of forty-six patients was compared to that of a control group of fifty-one patients. Patients in the control group were told nothing about postoperative pain; they were simply left to their imaginations and fears—their old meanings. The differences were striking. The patients in the special-care group were able to reduce their postoperative narcotic requirements by *half*. They also spent less time in the hospital, being discharged by their surgeons almost *three days earlier* than the control patients. (The surgeons did not know which patients were in which group, so they could not have steered the study in either direction; only the anesthesiologists knew who was receiving instructions.)

Even though the approach may seem intellectual, employing verbal information, it functioned at an emotional level. Much of the mystery of "having surgery" and the fear of the unknown were eliminated. The patients knew what to expect, and they did not feel helpless. The advice provided them with a sense of control over their pain: there was something *they* could do. But "control" does not describe the process fully, for in some sense the patients' control was attained only by letting go—letting the old meanings fall away, including dread, fear, and the expectation of pain.

Today modern hospitals are pushed to discharge patients "on time" by legislation that penalizes hospitals and physicians if hospital stays extend beyond a certain deadline. Enormous pressure is also exerted on physicians by the federal government and private insurance companies. Whether the policy of limiting hospital stays is a good or bad idea is not the issue here; what is of interest is that Egbert's study shows how this goal can be more easily accomplished. Honesty, a bit of time, a few words and caring are all that is required—no fancy equipment, expensive gadgets, or financial outlays. These simple measures allow *all* parties to be winners: the patient has a surgical experience that is humanized, experiences less pain and requires fewer drugs, and recovers more rapidly; the costs to the hospital are reduced; the surgeon has the gratification that the patient has done well and has experienced less pain, and his or her work load is reduced; and the federal government and the insurance company have spent less money.

Patients undergoing anesthesia should not assume that their surgeon or anesthesiologist will automatically employ these behavioral interventions. You must inquire and be prepared to give specific instructions to the health care team ahead of time if needed.

Hypnosis

Hypnosis is closely related to behavioral measures and is one of the oldest and best known mind-body therapies. It was used as early as 1821, when the French physician Recamier performed surgery on "magnetized" patients (at that time hypnotic phenomena were attributed to the influence of magnetized objects).

The appeal of hypnosis is enormous: it can be stunningly effective; it does not involve the use of drugs; and it allows patients to be conscious during a procedure, adding to their sense of control. In addition, hypnosis helps quell apprehension and anticipatory anxiety, increases tolerance to adverse stimuli, and intensifies whatever positive imagery the patient may be using at the time. It is quite compatible with many other techniques such as imagery, visualization, relaxation, and meditation. It has a wide range of applicability—diagnostic tests, surgery, the pain of acute or chronic illness, and rehabilitation.

Hypnosis makes possible a profound change of the meaning of medical experiences. By allowing a patient to remain conscious, it helps him or her retain a sense of participation and control. It helps counteract the passive, dependent, and helpless feelings that many persons find disempowering.[10]

But hypnosis isn't for everyone. Most people still have implicit faith in their health care team and are perfectly happy to trust the surgeon, anesthesiologist, and nurses to "do the right thing." They are not concerned with "retaining control" or "participating" in medical events. This is the "wake me when it's over" approach, and it is highly effective for most patients.

Which approach is best for you? Many books and publications can help you decide. One of the best sources of information for laypersons is the Institute for the Advancement of Health in San Francisco. This organization can provide monographs and articles on hypnosis, as well as on most of the other methods discussed in this section that can change meanings of health and illness.[11]

If you find hypnosis appealing, you can learn to be hypnotized or you can become considerably skilled in self-hypnosis with relatively little instruction. This is a marvelous skill to carry to the hospital. Today there are many therapists who are competent teachers of these techniques; ask your personal physician for some referrals.

Biofeedback, Imagery, and Visualization

One of the best nondrug methods of dealing with the pain and anxiety of any hospital experience is biofeedback. In biofeedback training, you work with a therapist and electronic devices that measure the pulse, skin temperature, or other indexes of anxiety. This information is "fed back" to conscious awareness via a meter or sound, so that you gradually gain purposeful control over the body's alarm reactions, which usually are not perceived until out of control. As you learn this skill (usually in a half-dozen sessions or less), you can "practice" the upcoming procedure by mentally rehearsing it through imagery and visualization, keeping the body's reactions under control all the while. Once mastered, this skill can be used outside the hospital setting in the everyday world. In addition to biofeedback, many other relaxation techniques are available, including self-hypnosis, already mentioned, and various meditation techniques, for which formal instruction is readily available.

Again, competent therapists are common, but there are also incompetent therapists. Be critical. Inquire about credentials. One of the best qualifications is certification by the Biofeedback Certification Institute of America.

The Guided Tour

Not only is it important to visit the room where you will be hospitalized, it can also be helpful to have a guided tour of the area of the hospital where your laboratory procedure will be done. (It generally will not be possible to tour surgery areas ahead of time because of sterility precautions.) Without being obtrusive or interfering, you can ask to meet the physicians, nurses, and technicians who will be present during the procedure. Familiarity with the surroundings and personnel helps remove fear of the unknown. So, too, does knowledge of the technical aspects of the upcoming procedure. Many diagnostic departments have written materials and/or audiotapes and videotapes that provide descriptions and other information. In addition, bookstores and libraries have a wide variety of home medical guides for laypersons, which detail almost all modern procedures. You will also want to ask whether the diagnostic department takes measures to help calm patients during the procedure, such as playing preselected music of the patient's choice, as mentioned above.

Fellow Patients

It can help enormously to talk with someone who has already been hospitalized for the same reason, or who has undergone the test for which you are scheduled—someone who has "been there." There is evidence that for some persons this sort of patient-to-patient communication is more effective at teaching and at allaying anxiety than any other measure. But one has to choose wisely who to talk to; some patients like to emphasize or exaggerate the risky nature of the procedure, as if to accentuate their own heroism for having made it through.

Qualifications

Another important question is who is to perform your tests in the hospital or who will be involved with surgery. Many persons place immense trust in their primary physician's decision on these matters, but for some this is not enough. They may realize that the incidence of side effects associated with medical acts vary widely. To know that a particular diagnostician has an admirable safety record can be reassuring. If uncertainty exists, it is best to directly ask one's doctor about the safety record of both the facility doing the testing and the diagnostician. If the answers aren't satisfying, it is probably best to inquire about other arrangements.

PUTTING IT ALL TOGETHER

Ellen, a fifty-five-year-old businesswoman, had experienced persistent uterine bleeding for two years. The problem could not be controlled with medications, and the blood loss was so severe it was a threat to her health. I referred her to a gynecologic surgeon, who advised a hysterectomy to solve the problem.

Because she had already tried every conservative solution, Ellen faced surgery with a calm resolve. She was in my office for her final presurgery visit, and we discussed her strategy for entering the hospital.

"I'm making a nuisance of myself," she informed me. "The admission clerks hate me. I've demanded a private room with the best possible view. They said they couldn't guarantee the room I wanted, but when I stood firm they changed their minds and relented. I don't like being pushy, but these things are important to me."

She went on to describe her visits to her surgeon, a skillful, kind gynecologist who supported her personal involvement in the preoperative decision making. Her anesthesiologist, however, was not as understanding.

"He had a bit of trouble at first with my requests," Ellen said. "I gave him a tape to play to me through my Walkman headphones during anesthesia. I also gave him some healing suggestions to speak to me before I awaken. He obviously had not been asked to do this before. At first he said playing the tape would interfere with anesthesia, and that he'd be too busy 'recovering' me to relay the suggestions. When I asked him for a referral to a colleague who might feel otherwise, he became much more interested and agreed that he could manage my requests. We came to a cordial agreement. I like him; he just needs a bit more training!"

The night before surgery Ellen checked into the hospital. I went by to see her on evening rounds. On entering her room I was startled. In one corner stood an easel with a large painting of a pastoral scene she had brought from home. On a corner table was a CD player, with speakers on either side. A striking floral arrangement graced a bedside stand. Instead of the usual white hospital linens, her bed was arrayed in her own colorful sheets, and an intricately designed homemade quilt lay at her feet.

"I'll be back in a moment," I stammered. "I need to check your lab work."

I went to the central nurses' station a short distance down the hall. While thumbing through her chart I noticed a large bowl of fruit between the computers on the secretarial work space. One of the nurses saw my puzzlement.

"Ellen, your patient, sent it," she said, "with thanks for our care. Sort of unusual: the thank-you gift arrived before *she* did."

Returning to her room, I found the lights dimmed. Ellen was listening to her audiocassette player through headphones.

"Nice accommodations," I remarked.

"Think I'm overdoing it?"

"Of course not. Anything that helps you get well is O.K. By the way, the thank-you gift for the nurses was a nice gesture. You've got their attention. You're not 'the hysterectomy in room 12'; already you're on a first-name basis."

Ellen's surgery the next morning was uneventful. All her presurgery requests were carried out smoothly, and her postoperative course was uncomplicated. She required almost no pain medication and left the hospital three days earlier than average.

In spite of the fact that she did not need my attention, I found myself visiting Ellen's room frequently. I suddenly realized that it simply was a pleasure to do so. Entering her room was uplifting—the art, music, and flowers were an oasis in the sterile environment of the hospital. My response was not unique. The nurses hovered over her continually. They, too, were affected by this unique woman who wanted to take part in her own healing.

Ellen's concerns that she would be viewed as an eccentric trouble-maker proved unfounded. Her vigorous persistence was in fact honored by the health care staff. They seemed to acknowledge her right to chart her own course and control her own experience. They found it refreshing to associate with her, to care for her, to be in her presence. Her effect on them lingered. Months later, long after she had left the hospital, the nurses who had cared for her continued casually to inquire, "How's Ellen?" Ellen not only had had a positive effect on her own health; she created a positive effect on "the system" as well.

Because there are not yet enough Planetree units to go around, we must individually do what we can to create our own. This does not mean we can restructure the entire hospital, but we can develop the skills we will need ahead of time, and communicate honestly and sincerely with the hospital personnel and physicians with whom we will be dealing. Often, the simple fact that health care professionals know you are critical and actively involved will get you kid-glove care.

TWENTY-TWO

Pictures in the Mind:
Using the Imagination
for Healing

It was Christmas Eve and Stephen was awaiting the amputation of his left foot. Three days earlier he had been Christmas shopping in a local mall. As he was returning to his car, laden with presents, a vehicle backed into him, pinning his left knee between two bumpers and crushing both the bones in the lower leg. He was rushed to the hospital, where the bones were set. Within hours, however, ominous signs appeared—dark discoloration of the left foot, with massive swelling and disappearance of all pulses from the knee downward. Stephen's foot was in trouble: the blood supply was being choked by the trauma to the arteries around the knee and the pressure from the swelling in the lower leg.

Following an arteriogram, which showed the site of the obstruction in the blood supply, Stephen's vascular surgeon performed a bypass operation, shunting blood around the damaged blood vessels to the leg below. Later a fasciotomy was done—an operation in which the rigid, tendonlike sheaths in the lower leg were severed—to relieve the pressure on the compressed vessels and enhance blood flow. Nothing worked. The foot was becoming darker, more swollen, and painful. Without a miracle, it would soon be amputated.

Angela, a cardiovascular nurse, had just been assigned to take care of Stephen. The nurse who had been caring for him told Angela that he was utterly unmanageable—angry, threshing about in bed, completely uncooperative, bordering on violence. She was glad to be going off duty; she was afraid of Stephen. He was six-four, weighed 240 pounds, and drove sixteen-wheelers coast to coast. His favorite sport was arm wrestling in roadside truckstops—contests that, as he put it, he "usually won."

During her initial bedside assessment Angela found that Stephen had already begun to describe his left leg as dead, detached from his body. He felt hopeless and confessed that he was very afraid.

Angela asked Stephen to participate in some simple in-bed relaxation techniques. He refused to, saying, "What's the use?" She kept asking him anyway, and finally he began to cooperate. His previous hostility seemed to melt. She asked him if he'd ever made pictures in his mind. "All the time," he replied. "Every time I arm wrestle at a truck stop I imagine my arm, shoulder, and upper body are made of steel that nobody can bend."

Angela measured the blood pressure in both lower legs with a Doppler device, a sensitive instrument that amplifies the sound of blood coursing through blood vessels. In his right foot the sound came through with a strong "swoosh," but it was completely absent on the left.

Then the nurse adjusted the device so that Stephen could himself listen to the loud swooshing of the blood flowing through the arteries in his normal right foot. She asked him to make a mental image of the sound.

"That's easy," he said. "It's a long hollow tube with blood flowing all the way to the toes." Stephen, the truck driver, hauled steel pipe.

Angela remained with him, guiding and coaxing him in making increasingly vivid pictures in the mind. After fifteen minutes she placed the Doppler device over the artery in the dark, swollen left foot.

"Hear anything?" she asked.

Stephen was speechless. Finally he managed, "Yes!"

Angela listened too. There was no mistaking the sound: Stephen's blood flow was returning. As she later said, "That moment was magical. I looked at Stephen; we both had tears in our eyes."

She left his bedside, and Stephen continued to exercise his mental imagery and relaxation. Now he needed no encouragement: he was fighting to save his foot, and it was working. Within a couple of hours his foot was warmer and pinker, and the pulses had actually become palpable. Stephen's leg was alive.

When his surgeon came by to discuss the amputation, he could not believe the change. He ascribed the improvement to the arterial bypass operation and fasciotomy done earlier—a "delayed effect," he said. Stephen explained what happened after the imagery, but his physician didn't buy it: this was a "physical problem." Still shaking his head in disbelief, he reached for the bedside phone, called the operating room, and removed Stephen from the surgery schedule.

It was time for change-of-shift. Before she left, Angela had one final conversation with Stephen. He wanted to know what had worked—the surgical procedures or the relaxation and imagery.

"I don't know for sure," she said. "Sometimes it takes both approaches. Remember: you have a lot of control over your own blood flow. Keep up the good work!" Stephen needed no reminders. A few days later he left the hospital, both feet intact.

Would blood flow have returned to Stephen's foot without imagery and relaxation? As Angela suggested, it is impossible to know. The point is that in uncertain situations it is important to take advantage of all possible forms of therapy, especially if there is a strong rationale for a new therapy and if it has no side effects.

For the past twenty years, research in biofeedback has shown that one can exert voluntary control over blood flow in certain areas of the body. This is particularly true in the vessels of the extremities, which are exquisitely sensitive to "pictures in the mind" because of a rich network of nerves leading to them from the brain. In addition they are responsive to chemicals such as adrenaline, a constrictor of blood vessels, whose concentration in the blood is in turn responsive to thoughts and emotions, diminishing during relaxation. Postulating that we can consciously participate in how our blood vessels behave is consistent with known principles of physiology and fits with observed facts. Stephen's case shows that to some extent the behavior of our blood vessels can be brought under the influence of our mind. So does the following case:

The woman sat across the physician's desk with her hands hidden. They were tucked out of sight under her dress, and she was half-sitting on them. They were the reason she had come.

Anna had Raynaud's disease, a common disorder of unknown cause in which the small blood vessels in the hands undergo constriction, choking off the blood supply. When the blood vessels go into spasm, the fingers can quite suddenly turn white as chalk, especially on exposure to cold, and at other times become red or purplish. These swings in color reflect changes in the amount of blood reaching the fingers and can be quite painful. When the blood supply suddenly diminishes, the fingers can become numb and coordination can be affected. The hands are usually cold and clammy at all times, which can be an unending source of embarrassment. The diminished blood supply can lead to ugly changes in the skin and nails. In this respect Anna was typical. She was so ashamed of her hands that she had not responded to the physician's offer of a handshake.

Raynaud's disease can be associated with a variety of other disorders, many of which are quite serious. However, extensive tests by previous physicians had failed to turn up any other problems with Anna.

The conversation between Anna and her physician was matter-of-fact. She was reluctant to divulge much about herself, wanting to focus only on her main concern, her painful, unsightly hands. After reviewing her medical records, the doctor referred her for biofeedback therapy as treatment for her problem.

Biofeedback had been shown conclusively to benefit patients with this condition and is a skill that is easily learned by most persons. During biofeedback the temperature of the hands is measured by exquisitely sensitive thermistors applied to the tips of the fingers. The temperature of the fingers is directly related to the amount of blood entering them. This information is then displayed on the biofeedback instruments for the patient to see, allowing awareness of a normally unconscious process. The goal is to increase the warmth of the fingers, and thus the amount of blood entering them. It is quite difficult to describe how anyone actually accomplishes this—as difficult, perhaps, as describing how one rides a bicycle. Yet the skill is not difficult to learn and becomes so natural that it eventually is intuitive and automatic. At this point, the "gadgets" aren't necessary, and patients can transfer this ability into everyday life. [1]

Anna, like most patients encountering biofeedback for the first time, was skeptical. She had little confidence and wasn't sure biofeedback would work, despite the fact that it had helped many other people with her problem. She was even more taken aback when Beth, the biofeedback therapist, asked her on her first visit, "Draw your hands for me."

"I thought I came here for biofeedback training, not *art* lessons," she responded coolly.

"That's right," Beth said patiently. "But I want to know the pictures in your mind. That will give us both some idea about what your hands *mean* to you."

"What's *that* got to do with my problem?" Anna demanded.

With some encouragement she complied. She drew ugly hands with the crayons—fat and misshapen, with thick, clubbed fingers. These were not human hands. The fingers were like bark, with flaking skin projecting from them like shards. The only color she used on this grotesque and angry image was black.

In just a few sessions Anna mastered biofeedback training. Her hand temperature began in the truly frigid range, 65 degrees Fahrenheit, and increased into the mid-90s by her fourth session. Eventually she discovered that the instruments were not necessary. She could warm her hands without them, and she began to do so even outside the biofeedback laboratory. During the process her symptoms totally abated. Slowly, the physical appearance of her hands changed. They became normally pink and warm, and her nails regained a normal texture and shape. She no longer kept them tucked under her dress or behind her back, and she had even begun to initiate handshaking.

On her last session she was jubilant about her success. Once again Beth took out the art pad. "Would you draw what your hands mean to you now?" she asked.

This time Anna did not object. Now her drawing was radically different—long, slender, pink fingers with beautiful, perfect nails. The fingers were adorned with rings she had begun to wear again, jewelry unused for the years her problem had existed. These were human hands now, and they belonged to a person who was obviously very proud of them.

Beth retrieved her initial drawing from her file and placed it beside the new one. Seeing the contrast, Anna began to smile. Then the smile vanished and she became pensive, and tears formed. Staring at the before-and-after drawings, she turned to Beth.

"I can't thank you enough for what you've done for me," she said.

"I haven't done much. It's you who has done the work. I've just been your guide. But could you tell me what your hands mean to you now?"

Anna related how her entire life had taken different directions as her hands had changed. No longer were they a symbol of disease, despair, inadequacy, and ugliness. Now they were a part of her total body, which she was proud to own. As she felt her self-image transforming, she experienced phenomenal shifts in her level of confidence. This had led to changes in her job performance and in her relationships with others.

"This was not just 'hand problems'," she allowed. "My hands represented my whole life. When they changed, my life changed. My hands were a mirror of my life."[2]

Anna had arrived at an uncommon level of understanding of her problem. The biofeedback training allowed her a sense of mastery over her physiology and was an important assist in overcoming her belief that her problem was "all physical." It helped her escape her victim mentality, her idea that she was essentially held hostage by her malfunctioning body.

Anna's experience suggests the rich variety of methods available today for achieving breakthroughs in many complex medical problems. These methods frequently are most effective when they are used together with counseling.

Often an imagery-based method such as biofeedback can be extraordinarily helpful because it gives a vivid demonstration of the interconnection of mind and body. One can literally see the ability of thoughts, emotions, and certain psychological strategies to move meters and trigger lights and sounds on the biofeedback instruments. This can be a meaning-rich experience for many persons, illustrating that the body is not fixed and immutable but can be shaped by one's own consciousness.

> Until 1933, no Rolls-Royce was equipped with a reverse gear. Sir Henry Royce was not willing for his car to have what he considered an undignified mode of progression.
>
> —CHARLES JOHNSON[3]

Some people seem to regard "using the mind" rather like Sir Henry viewed reverse gear—as somehow unbecoming. They may regard therapies that emphasize mental effort as archaic, superstitious, and unscientific. Yet many of these approaches, as evidenced by the impressive research in the field of biofeedback, have been proven scientifically to add another dimension to health care. Just as reverse gear does not take the place of the forward gears, mind-based strategies do not supplant physically based ones. Rather, they add a new dimension, a new capability, a means of going in new directions in the task of getting well.

Afterword

The medical tales we have examined so far have mainly involved dramatic, life-or-death events. But most of our health problems are not of this magnitude. They are mundane, banal, ordinary; they weigh us down and discourage us but do not send us to the emergency room, cancer ward, or coronary care unit. Yet meaning enters the simplest situations as resoundingly as it does the most serious health events, and can transform them just as profoundly. I want to close with a story of one of the commonest maladies—headache—and show that a change in meaning can free us from the curse of even the most ordinary problems.

Migraine headache is extraordinarily common and comes in many varieties and levels of severity. At its worst it can be unbearable: people have committed suicide to escape it. At age fourteen, I began to be troubled with severe migraine headaches. My particular problem was the classic type—temporary blindness and "flashing lights" involving much of the field of vision, agonizing headache, and intractable nausea and vomiting, followed by twenty-four hours of near-incapacitation. Through the years I went to physicians, who reassured me it was "only" migraine and nothing worse, such as a brain tumor, in which case, they told me, I'd already be dead. None of this was any comfort. The myriad medications I tried failed to work, and I decided I simply was stuck with the problem.

During medical school the syndrome began to trouble me in another way. I became concerned that sooner or later I would experience a typical episode of partial blindness, nausea, and vomiting in a life-or-death setting such as a medical emergency or surgery. Other physicians might not be around to bail me out. Because I could not possibly function well in these situations, I realized I would be putting a patient's life at risk. I also knew that I had not disclosed this problem on my application to medical school, and I began to fear it was only a matter of time until I was discovered. The problem therefore took on ethical dimensions. Since I'd already tried every therapy I'd ever heard of to no avail, the only solution I could think of was simply to drop out of medical school.

I made an appointment to see Dr. James, my faculty adviser, to inform him of my decision. He was the retiring chairman of the department of pediatrics and a physician of the old school—gentlemanly, avuncular, urbane, sensitive, and eminently kind. Dr. James could see I was deeply troubled. His patience and concern surprised me, for I'd expected criticism for not revealing my problem on my medical school application. When I finished there was a period of silence while I waited for the worst.

Finally he said slowly with a gentle smile, "I think you should do nothing and just relax."

I was stunned. What novel suggestions! *Never* had I considered relaxing, let alone doing nothing.

"When I was young," he continued, "I, too, had migraine headaches. They went away, which is typical as one gets older. Even if you do nothing, your headaches will get much better, so there is nothing to worry about. Above all you must stay in medical school. It is the only thing to do."

By this time my mind was a blur. I cannot remember what, if anything, I offered in response, and I left in complete confusion.

Dr. James was wrong. My headaches did not get better but continued much as before. But it no longer mattered, for now the entire problem *seemed* different. Dr. James had given me *hope,* the expectation and belief that things would improve. He had not manipulated my illness but only the *meaning* it contained for me. I do not mean that I embraced migraine headaches thereafter; I would have preferred they disappear (as they practically did years later when I discovered biofeedback as an intervention for the problem). Yet my response went beyond merely being hopeful. A new relationship with my problem slowly developed, as the psychological distance between migraine and me diminished. I began to regard it not as something I *had* but as something I *was*. These new meanings helped me keep my career on track.

The wise old pediatrician had functioned as a "meaning therapist." With only a few words he taught me not a new way of *doing* but a different way of *being*—the hallmark of all "meaning therapy." At that time the concept of meaning was hardly in my vocabulary, let alone my life. But even though I could not articulate what happened, I experienced firsthand the power of meaning to transform disease and diminish its toll, *even though the pathology remained.*

During the last century, the American physician Oliver Wendell Holmes observed that

> there is nothing men will not do, there is nothing they have not done to recover their health and save their lives. They have submitted to be half-drowned in water, and half-choked with gases, to be buried up to their chins in earth, to be seared with hot irons like galley-slaves, to be crimped with knives like codfish, to swallow all sorts of abominations, and to pay for all this, as if to be singed and scalded were a costly privilege, as if blisters were a blessing and leeches a luxury. What more can be asked to prove their honesty and sincerity?[1]

Holmes, who was a gifted and compassionate physician, was not poking fun. His description is poignant: the desperation and fear that people sense when seriously sick will drive them to any length in search of a cure. Although some of the approaches Holmes described have been replaced by scientific therapies, our stop-at-nothing efforts to restore health have not changed. In my own life and work I honor these physical approaches to health care. But in this book I have wanted also to show that *whatever* external approaches we choose, disease has another side, which can be approached not through *doing* but through *understanding*. Illness contains an inner code by which it wants to "say something," a silent language through which it frequently symbolizes or represents a variety of "invisibles," as E. F. Schumacher called them. We have called these invisibles *meanings*.

Sometimes they bubble up from our unconscious and float to the surface of the mind, and we "catch the meaning" of an illness-event. Moreover, as the stories in this book show, our own perceived meanings enter the body and actually change it for better or worse, and become part of the inner code of meaning.

But with our limited ways of knowing, it is not always possible to understand the role of meaning in any given health-event. In view of these limitations, perhaps our task is simply to be open to meaning, not just in illness but in *all* adversity—to be receptive, to seek whatever wisdom life's difficult moments may convey, to honor whatever mystery they may contain. Rainer Maria Rilke, the great German poet, expressed this attitude in his *Letters to a Young Poet*—which I often have thought could appropriately be called *Letters to a Young Doctor:*

> Why do you want to shut out of your life any agitation, any pain, any melancholy, since you really do not know what these states are working upon you? . . . If there is anything morbid in your processes, just remember that sickness is the means by which an organism frees itself of foreign matter; so one must just help it to be sick, to have its whole sickness and break out with it, for that is its progress.[2]

Our journey into meaning hopefully will always continue, for that is the path of our humanness. My wish is that these medical tales will aid each reader in the search for his or her own meanings—a search that, if successful, will return always to the epigraph of this book:

Meaning is being.

Notes

Epigraph, p. vii: David Bohm, "Meaning and Information," in *The Search for Meaning*, Paavo Pylkkänen, ed. (Wellingborough, Northamptonshire, England: Crucible, 1989), p. 51.

ACKNOWLEDGMENTS

1. Larry Dossey, *Space, Time & Medicine* (Boston: Shambhala, 1982).
2. D. S. Kothari, "Atom and Self," the Meghnad Saha Medal Lecture—1978, *Proceedings of the Indian National Science Academy*, Part A, Physical Science 46:1 (1980), pp. 1–28.

INTRODUCTION

1. Nikos Kazantzakis, *Zorba the Greek* (New York: Simon & Schuster, 1952), p. 45.
2. Myiasis merited inclusion in one of the strangest books I have ever come across, written by Philadelphia physicians George M. Gould and Walter L. Pyle and published in 1896, *Anomalies and Curiosities of Medicine—Being an encyclopedic collection of rare and extraordinary cases, and of the most striking instances of abnormality in all branches of medicine and surgery, derived from an exhaustive research of medical literature from its origin to the present day, abstracted, classified, annotated, and indexed* (!). (An adaptation of this book has been republished recently by

Hammond Publishing Company as *Medical Curiosities*.) After noting the "not uncommon" occurrence of myiasis around the world, the authors describe the experience of Indian surgeons with it. "Worms lodging in the cribriform plate of the ethmoid [sinus areas of the nose] feed on the soft tissues of that region. Eventually their ravages destroy the olfactory nerves, with subsequent loss of the sense of smell, and they finally eat away the bridge of the nose. The head of the victim droops, and he complains of crawling of worms in the interior of the nose. The eyelids swell so that the patient cannot see, and a deformity arises which exceeds that produced by syphilis." Thus was a Dr. Lyons, writing in the *Indian Annals of Medicine,* October 1885, moved to state that myiasis "is one of the most loathsome diseases that comes under the observation of medical men."

One of the most famous American cases dates to 1883 and was originally reported in the *Medical Monthly* of Peoria, Illinois, by a Dr. Richardson. A traveler in Kansas was sleeping when a fly laid its eggs in its nose, "probably attracted by a discharge of mucus." The first symptoms were those of a severe cold. As the maggots cut away through the tissues, the man became delirious and complained of intense misery and annoyance in the nose and head. The worms finally bored through the soft palate, impairing his speech, and moved on to the eustachian tubes. Although the surgeon was able to remove 250 maggots, the man eventually died. (Reported in Richard Wall and Jamie Stevens, "The Turn of the Screw Worm," *New Scientist,* June 9, 1990, pp. 54–57.)

3. Mircea Eliade, *The Sacred and the Profane* (San Diego: Harcourt Brace Jovanovich, 1959), p. 165.

4. *Webster's New Collegiate Dictionary* (Springfield, MA: G. & C. Merriam Co., 1959), p. 520.

5. E. F. Schumacher, *A Guide for the Perplexed* (New York: Harper & Row, 1977), p. 35.

6. T. S. Eliot, "Choruses From 'The Rock,'" *Selected Poems* (New York: Harvest/Harcourt Brace Jovanovich, 1964), p. 107.

7. Archibald MacLeish, quoted in Rollo May, *Paulus: Tillich as Spiritual Teacher* (Dallas: Saybrook, 1988), p. 118.

8. Arthur J. Deikman, "Sufism and the Mental Health Sciences," in R. Walsh and D. H. Shapiro, eds., *Beyond Health and Normality* (New York: Van Nostrand Reinhold, 1983), p. 275.

9. Sigmund Freud, quoted in Michael Polanyi, *Personal Knowledge* (Chicago: University of Chicago Press, 1962), p. 233.

10. Freeman Dyson, *Disturbing the Universe* (New York: Harper & Row, 1979), p. 249.

11. David Bohm, quoted in *Bulletin of the Foundation for Mind-Being Research,* September 1988, p. 3.

12. Paul Davies, *The Cosmic Blueprint* (New York: Simon & Schuster, 1989), p. 203.

13. Personal communication from Paul Anderson, M.D., January 1986.

14. Alfred Korzybski, lecture to seminar, 1951, quoted in Lawrence LeShan, *The Dilemma of Psychology* (New York: Dutton, 1990), p. 74.

15. Ellen L. Idler and Stanislav Kasl, "Health Perceptions and Survival: Do

Global Evaluations of Health Status Really Predict Mortality?" *Journal of Gerontology* 46:2 (1991) S55–65.

16. Daniel Goleman, "Mortality Study Lends Weight to Patient's Opinion," *The New York Times* March 21, 1991, p. B13.

17. Ibid., p. B13.

18. There is another possibility why one's opinion of his of her health is a potent predictor of mortality for all age groups. People may simply have the capacity to know the future, including their own life-or-death. This possibility is currently so foreign to science that it is not even mentioned by the researchers who conducted the above studies. Yet we cannot discount this possibility, especially in view of the experimental evidence favoring it. Many experiments have demonstrated that there is some aspect of the human psyche that is *nonlocal*—unconfined to points in space, such as brains or bodies, or to points in time, such as the present moment. Such a mental faculty would permit people to scan ahead to know directly what awaits them, and to return to the present with an opinion about their state of health. For a summary of this evidence, see Larry Dossey, *Recovering the Soul* (New York: Bantam, 1991).

19. Susan Sontag, *Illness as Metaphor* (New York: Farrar, Straus and Giroux, 1977).

20. Alfred North Whitehead, quoted in T. S. Ananthu, *Science Dynamics: A Newly Emerging Paradigm* (New Dehli: Gandhi Peace Foundation, 1987), p. 21.

21. The rationale for meaninglessness in persons schooled in science is frequently that the universe is simply too vast and complex to "care" and we are too insignificant to make a difference. This view was expressed by novelist Stephen Crane (1871–1900): "A man said to the universe, 'Sir, I exist.' The universe said, 'However, the fact has not created in me a sense of obligation.'"

22. C. G. Jung, *Memories, Dreams, Reflections*, Aniela Jaffé, ed., Richard Winston and Clara Winston, trans. (New York: Vintage, 1965), p. 340.

23. Eugene P. Wigner, "Are We Machines?" *Proceedings of the American Philosophical Society* 113:2 (1969), pp. 95–101.

PART ONE, BREAKDOWN

1. Albert Einstein, *Ideas and Opinions* (New York: Crown, 1954), p. 11.

2. C. G. Jung, *Psychology and the Occult* (Princeton: Princeton University Press, 1977), pp. 136–137.

1, THE ASTHMATIC AND THE INTERN:
WHEN SHAME IS FATAL

1. Adapted from James J. Lynch, *The Broken Heart: The Medical Consequences of Loneliness* (New York: Basic Books, 1977), pp. 111–112 (case originally reported in Julius Bauer, "Sudden, Unexpected Death," *Postgraduate Medicine* 22 [1957], pp. A34–A35).

2. Barrie Cassileth, B. R. Cassileth, E. J. Lusk, T. B. Strouse, and B. J. Bodenheimer, "Contemporary Unorthodox Treatments in Cancer Medicine: A Study of Patients, Treatments, and Practitioners," *Annals of Internal Medicine* 10 (1984), pp. 105–112.

3. Joan Borysenko, *Guilt Is the Teacher, Love Is the Lesson* (New York: Warner, 1990), pp. 26 ff.

4. Blair Justice, *Who Gets Sick: Thinking and Health* (Houston: Peak Press, 1987), pp. 230–231. Reprinted as *Who Gets Sick: How Beliefs, Moods and Thoughts Affect Your Health* (Los Angeles: J. P. Tarcher, 1988). All subsequent references refer to the Peak Press edition.

5. Shelley E. Taylor, *Positive Illusions: Creative Self-Deception and the Healthy Mind* (New York: Basic Books, 1989), pp. 187–188.

6. Martin E. P. Seligman, "Helplessness and Explanatory Style: Risk Factors for Depression and Disease," paper presented at the annual meeting of the Society of Behavioral Medicine, San Francisco, March 1986; quoted in Justice, op. cit., pp. 229–230.

2, CAUGHT IN THE ACT:
FORBIDDEN PLAY AND CARDIAC ARREST

1. Adapted from Bernard Lown et al., "Basis for Recurring Ventricular Fibrillation in the Absence of Coronary Heart Disease and Its Management," *New England Journal of Medicine* 294:12 (1976), pp. 623–629. (Dr. Lown is sometimes credited with being "the inventor of the defibrillator." However, crude versions of defibrillators have been around for a century and can be viewed at a remarkable museum and library, the Bakken, in Minneapolis, Minnesota. This institution was established by Earl Bakken, who invented the implantable cardiac pacemaker, and is dedicated to exploring the uses of electricity in health and healing through the ages.)

2. Martin S. Gizzi and Bernard Gitler, "Coronary Risk Factors: The Contemplation of Bigamy," letter to the editor, *Journal of the American Medical Association* 256:9 (1986), p. 1138.

3. J. B. Morgagni, *The Seats and Causes of Diseases,* vol. I, Benjamin Alexander trans. (London: Millar and Cadell, 1769), pp. 795 ff. See Ralph H. Major, *Classic Descriptions of Disease* (Springfield, IL: Charles C. Thomas, 1945), pp. 450–452. See also Fielding H. Garrison, *History of Medicine,* 4th ed. (Philadelphia: W. B. Saunders, 1929), pp. 353–354.

4. M. Ueno, "The So-called Coition Death," *Japan Journal of Legal Medicine* 17 (1963), p. 330. See T. P. Hackett and J. F. Rosenbaum, "Emotion, Psychiatric Disorders, and the Heart," in E. Braunwald, ed., *Heart Disease* (Philadelphia: W. B. Saunders, 1980), pp. 1923 ff.

5. Joan Borysenko, *Guilt Is the Teacher, Love Is the Lesson* (New York: Warner, 1990), p. 28.

6. Blair Justice, *Who Gets Sick: Thinking and Health* (Houston: Peak Press, 1987), p. 216.

3. THE SIEGE OF SHAME:
THE MULTIPLE PERSONALITY DISORDER

1. Judith Hooper and Dick Teresi, *The Three-Pound Universe* (New York: Dell, 1986), p. 241.
2. Judith Hooper and Dick Teresi, "Mind Menagerie," *OMNI,* January 1986, pp. 74 ff.
3. Edward Dolnick, "The People Inside," *Hippocrates* 3:4 (1989), p. 39.
4. Joan Borysenko, *Guilt Is the Teacher, Love Is the Lesson* (New York: Warner, 1990), p. 53.
5. Frank Putnam quoted in Edward Dolnick, op. cit., p. 39.
6. Hooper and Teresi, *The Three-Pound Universe,* p. 241.
7. Bruno Bettelheim quoted in Edward Dolnick, op. cit., p. 39.
8. Hooper and Teresi, "Mind Menagerie," p. 104.
9. D. R. Weinberger, R. L. Wagner, and R. J. Wyatt, "Neuropathological Studies of Schizophrenia: A Selected Review," *Schizophrenia Bulletin* 9, pp. 193–212. See also Frank Putnam, *Diagnosis and Treatment of Multiple Personality* (New York: Guilford, 1989).
10. Daniel Goleman, *Vital Lies, Simple Truths* (New York: Simon & Schuster, 1985), pp. 88–89.
11. Piero Ferrucci, *What We May Be: Techniques for Psychological and Spiritual Growth* (Los Angeles: J. P. Tarcher, 1982), pp. 47–48.
12. "Multiple Personality—Mirrors of a New Model of Mind?" *Investigations* (research bulletin of the Institute of Noetic Sciences) 1:¾, p. 9.
13. Ibid.
14. "Consciousness and Survival," *Newsletter of the Institute of Noetic Sciences* 13:3 (1985–1986), pp. 3–6.

4. HALLOWEEN AND HELPLESSNESS:
TO MEAN NOTHING IS TO DIE

1. Adapted from W. A. Greene, S. Goldstein, and A. J. Moss, "Psychological Aspects of Sudden Death," *Archives of Internal Medicine* 129 (1972), pp. 725–731.
2. Bernard Lown et al., "Psychophysiological Factors in Sudden Cardiac Death," *American Journal of Psychiatry* 137:11 (1980), pp. 1325–1335.
3. George L. Engel, "Sudden and Rapid Death during Psychological Stress: Folklore or Folk Wisdom?" *Annals of Internal Medicine* 74 (1971), pp. 771–782.
4. Ibid., p. 773.
5. "Low Death Rate for Jewish Men at Passover Shows Will to Live," *Brain/Mind Bulletin* 14:4 (1989), p. 4.
6. J. C. Coolidge, "Unexpected Death in a Patient Who Wished to Die," *Journal of the American Psychoanalytical Association* 17 (1969), pp. 413–420.
7. L. J. Saul, "Sudden Death at Impasse," *Psychological Forum* 1 (1966), pp. 88–89.
8. Joel E. Dimsdale, "Emotional Causes of Sudden Death," *American Journal of Psychiatry* 134 (1977), pp. 1361–1366.

5, VOODOO DEATH:
THE "NO EXIT" SYNDROME

1. Walter Cannon, "Voodo Death," *American Anthropologist* 44 (1942), pp. 169–181.
2. Norman Cousins, "Belief Becomes Biology," *Advances* 6:3 (1989), pp. 20–29. See also Norman Cousins, *Head First: The Biology of Hope* (New York: E. P. Dutton, 1989).
3. William James, *Principles of Psychology* (New York: Longmans, Green and Co., 1905), pp. 179–180.
4. Cannon, op. cit., p. 182.
5. Ibid.
6. For an example of modern-day voodoo and how a countercharm was administered in a large modern hospital with lifesaving results, see "Hexes and Molecules" in my *Space, Time & Medicine* (Boston: New Science Library, 1982), pp. 3–8.
7. Ellen J. Langer and Judith Rodin, "The Effects of Choice and Enhanced Personal Responsibility for the Aged: A Field Experiment in an Institutional Setting," *Journal of Personality and Social Psychology* 34 (1976), pp. 191–198. See Blair Justice, "Taking Charge and Living Longer," in *Who Gets Sick: Thinking and Health* (Houston: Peak Press, 1987), pp. 141–172.

6, BLACK MONDAY SYNDROME:
WHEN DREAD MEANS DEAD

1. S. W. Rabkin, F. A. L. Mathewson, and R. B. Tate, "Chronobiology of Cardiac Sudden Death in Men," *Journal of the American Medical Association* 244:12 (1980), pp. 1357–1358. See also James E. Muller et al., "Circadian Variation in the Frequency of Sudden Death," *Circulation* 75 (January 1987), p. 131.
2. *Work in America: Report of a Special Task Force to the Secretary of Health, Education, and Welfare* (Cambridge, MA: MIT Press, 1973).
3. C. D. Jenkins, "Psychological and Social Precursors of Coronary Artery Disease," *New England Journal of Medicine* 284 (1971), pp. 244–255.
4. Gina Kolata, "Heart Attacks at 9:00 A.M.," *Science* 233 (July 25, 1986), pp. 417–418.
5. Ibid.
6. D. M. Spengler et al., "Back Injuries in Industry: A Retrospective Study—Overview and Cost Analysis, Injury Factors, and Employee-Related Factors," *Spine* 11:3 (1986), pp. 241–256.
7. Suzanne C. Kobasa, "Stressful Life Events, Personality, and Health: An Inquiry into Hardiness," *Journal of Personality and Social Psychology* 37:1 (1979), pp. 1–11, and Salvatore R. Maddi and Suzanne C. Kobasa, *The Hardy Executive: Health under Stress* (Homewood, IL: Dow Jones–Irwin, 1984). See also Chapter 8, "Getting Ahead and Getting Cancer," in this book for the results of Kobasa's studies on a group of attorneys subjected to job stresses.

8. Blair Justice, *Who Gets Sick: Thinking and Health* (Houston: Peak Press, 1987), p. 61.

9. D. C. McClelland, G. Ross, and V. Patel, "The Effect of an Academic Examination on Salivary Norepinephrine and Immunoglobin Levels," *Journal of Human Stress* 11:2 (1985), pp. 52–59.

10. For a review of the relevant studies done in this area, see Blair Justice, "Surviving War and Captivity," in *Who Gets Sick: Thinking and Health,* pp. 70–72.

11. Aaron Antonovsky, *Health, Stress, and Coping* (San Francisco: Josey-Bass, 1979).

12. W. T. Boyce, C. Schaefer, and C. Uitti, "Permanence and Change: Psychological Factors in the Outcome of Adolescent Pregnancy," *Social Science and Medicine* 21:1 (1985), pp. 1279–1287.

7, JOHNNY CAN'T READ, JOHNNY HAS HEART DISEASE: EDUCATION, ISOLATION, AND HEALTH

1. T. B. Graboys, "Stress and the Aching Heart," *New England Journal of Medicine* 311:9 (1984), pp. 594–595.

2. W. Ruberman et al., "Psychosocial Influences on Mortality after Myocardial Infarction," *New England Journal of Medicine* 311:9 (1984), pp. 552–559.

3. L. Berkman and S. Syme, "Social Networks, Host Resistance, and Mortality: A Nine-year Follow-up Study of Alameda County Residents," *American Journal of Epidemiology* 109 (1982), pp. 186–204.

4. J. House, C. Robbins, and H. Metzner, "The Association of Social Relationships and Activities with Mortality: Prospective Evidence from the Tecumseh Study," *American Journal of Epidemiology* 116 (1982), pp. 123–140. See also J. House, K. R. Landis, and D. Umberson, "Social Relationships and Health," *Science* 241 (1988), pp. 540–545.

5. Leonard A. Sagan, *The Health of Nations: True Causes of Sickness and Well-being* (New York: Basic Books, 1987), p. 141.

6. Ibid., p. 181.

7. Robert M. Sapolsky, "Stress in the Wild," *Scientific American,* January 1990, pp. 116–123.

8. C. D. Jenkins, "Psychological and Social Precursors of Coronary Disease," *New England Journal of Medicine* 284 (1971), pp. 244–255.

8, THE PATIENT PATIENT: THE HAZARDS OF THE MEDICAL EXPERIENCE

1. Adapted from R. Tizes, "Cardiac Arrest Following Routine Venipuncture," *Journal of the American Medical Association* 236 (1976), pp. 1846–1847.

2. Adapted from George L. Engel, "The Care of the Patient: Art or Science?" *Johns Hopkins Medical Journal* 140 (1977), pp. 222–232.

3. Adapted from Jon Kabat-Zinn, *Full Catastrophe Living: A Practical Guide to Mindfulness, Meditation, and Healing* (New York: Delacorte, 1990).

4. Personal communication, source anonymous, 1989.

5. Personal communication, source anonymous, 1984.

6. Anthony F. Lalli, "Contrast Media Reactions: Data Analysis and Hypothesis," *Radiology* 134 (1980), pp. 1–12.

7. Ibid., p. 1.

8. Ibid., p. 12. Thanks to Howard J. Barnhard, M.D., Department of Radiology, University of Arkansas Medical School, for calling my attention to the work of Dr. Anthony F. Lalli.

9, GETTING AHEAD AND GETTING CANCER: THE PROBLEMS OF BEING A MEDICAL STUDENT

1. Quoted in Henry K. Silver and Anita Duhl Glicken, "Medical Student Abuse: Incidence, Severity, and Significance," *Journal of the American Medical Association* 263:4 (1990), pp. 527–532.

2. Quoted in ibid., p. 530.

3. Quoted in ibid., p. 530.

4. K. H. Sheehan, D. V. Sheehan, K. White, A. Leibowitz, and DeW. C. Baldwin, "A Pilot Study of Medical Student 'Abuse': Student Perceptions of Mistreatment and Misconduct in Medical School," *Journal of the American Medical Association* 263:4 (1990), pp. 533–537. For a proposed solution see Mary Hornig-Rohan, "Making Medical Education Healthier: A Student's View," *Advances* 4:2 (1987), pp. 24–28.

5. Quoted in Richard Erodes, *Lame Deer: Seeker of Vision* (New York: Simon & Schuster, 1972), p. 159.

6. Caroline B. Thomas, "Precursors of Premature Disease and Death: The Predictive Potential of Habits and Family Attitudes," *Annals of Internal Medicine* 85 (1976), pp. 653–658.

7. The subject of medical student abuse is out of the closet and onto the table. See Silver and Glicken, op. cit., and Sheehan et al., op. cit.

8. Silver and Glicken, op. cit., p. 527.

9. J. C. Barefoot, W. G. Dahlstrom, and R. B. Williams, "Hostility, Coronary Heart Disease Incidence, and Total Mortality: A 25-Year Follow-up Study of 255 Physicians," *Psychosomatic Medicine* 45:1 (1983), pp. 59–63.

10. Suzanne C. Kobasa, "Commitment and Coping in Stress Resistance among Lawyers," *Journal of Personality and Social Psychology* 42:4 (1982), pp. 707–717.

11. Blair Justice, *Who Gets Sick: Thinking and Health* (Houston: Peak Press, 1987), p. 60

12. Viktor E. Frankl, *Man's Search for Meaning* (New York: Washington Square Press, 1963).

10. BROKEN HEARTS:
THE TOXICITY OF BEREAVEMENT

1. Tim Jeal, *Livingstone* (New York: Dell, 1973), p. 399.
2. This report appeared in E. Gurney, F. W. H. Myers, and F. Podmore, *Phantasms of the Living,* abridged ed. (London: Kegan, Paul, Trench, Trübner, 1918), pp. 132–133. More recently it appeared in Ian Stevenson, *Telepathic Impressions* (Charlottesville: University Press of Virginia, 1970), p. 109, and in Lawrence LeShan, *From Newton to ESP* (Wellingtonborough, Northamptonshire, England: Turnstone Press, 1984), pp. 22–24.
3. Adapted from Stevenson, op. cit., p. 55.
4. Adapted from ibid., pp. 105–107.
5. Steven J. Schleifer, S. E. Keller, M. Camerino, J. C. Thornton, and M. Stein, "Suppression of Lymphocyte Stimulation Following Bereavement," *Journal of the American Medical Association* 250:3 (1983), pp. 374–377.
6. T. H. Holmes and R. H. Rahe, "The Social Readjustment Rating Scale," *Journal of Psychosomatic Research* 11 (1967), pp. 213–218.
7. W. D. Rees and S. G. Lutkins, "Mortality of Bereavement," *British Medical Journal* 4 (1967), pp. 13–16.
8. James J. Lynch, *The Broken Heart: The Medical Consequences of Loneliness* (New York: Basic Books, 1977), p. 56. See also Joan B. Stoddard and James P. Henry, "Affectional Bonding and the Impact of Bereavement," *Advances* 2:2 (1985), pp. 19–28.
9. B. A. van der Kolk, "Psychobiology of Attachment/Separation," *Psychiatric Times/Medicine and Behavior,* April 1987, p. 4.
10. Ibid.
11. Lynch, op. cit., pp. 75–76. (Previously cited in Lytt I. Gardner, "Deprivation Dwarfism," *Scientific American* 227 (1972), pp. 76–82.
12. Schleifer et. al., op. cit.
13. R. W. Bartrop, E. Luckhurst, L. Lazarus, L. G. Kiloh, and R. Penny, "Depressed Lymphocyte Function after Bereavement," *Lancet* 1:8016 (1977), pp. 834–836.
14. J. K. Kiecolt-Glaser, W. Garner, C. Speicher, G. Penn, J. Holliday, and R. Glaser, "Psychosocial Modifiers of Immunocompetence in Medical Students," *Psychosomatic Medicine* 46:1 (1984), pp. 7–14.
15. L. Berkman and S. Syme, "Social Networks, Host Resistance, and Mortality: A Nine-Year Follow-up Study of Alameda County Residents," *American Journal of Epidemiology* 109 (1982), pp. 186–204. See also P. Reynolds and G. A. Kaplan, "Social Connections and Cancer: A Prospective Study of Alameda County Residents," paper presented at the annual meeting of the Society of Behavioral Medicine, San Francisco, March 1986.
16. Adapted from Lynch, op. cit., pp. 58–59. Originally reported in I. C. Wilson and J. C. Reece, "Stimultaneous Death in Schizophrenic Twins," *Archives of General Psychiatry* 11 (1964), pp. 377–384.
17. Larry Dossey, *Recovering the Soul* (New York: Bantam, 1989).

18. Erwin Schrödinger, *What Is Life? and Mind and Matter* (London: Cambridge University Press, 1969), p. 145.

PART TWO, NEW MEANING, NEW BODY

1. From the Foreword by John Archibald Wheeler, in John D. Barrow and Frank J. Tipler, *The Anthropic Cosmological Principle* (New York: Oxford University Press, 1986).

11, MEANING LINKS MIND AND MATTER: THE THEORY OF PHYSICIST DAVID BOHM

1. David Bohn, quoted in *Brain/Mind Bulletin* 10:10 (1985), pp. 1–2.
2. *Webster's New Universal Unabridged Dictionary* (New York: Dorset and Baber, 1983).
3. David Bohm, "The Theory of Soma-Significance," Personal communication, 1985. For a description of the theory, see David Bohm, "Meaning and Information," in Paavo Pylkkänen, *The Search for Meaning* (Wellingborough, Northamptonshire, England: Crucible, 1989), and David Bohm, "Soma Significance: A New Notion of the Relationship between the Physical and the Mental," in Donald Factor, ed., *Unfolding Meaning* (London: Routledge and Kegan Paul 1987), pp. 72–120.
4. Personal communication, op, cit., p. 4.
5. Personal communication, op. cit., pp. 25–26.
6. Alfred North Whitehead, *Modes of Thought* (New York: Macmillan, 1968), pp. 156–165.
7. Personal communication, op. cit., p. 11.
8. Gregory Bateson, quoted in Jeremy Hayward, *Perceiving Ordinary Magic* (Boston: New Science Library, 1985), p. 214.

12, THE BODY AS MACHINE

1. Julien Offray de La Mettrie, "Man: A Machine (London: G. Smith, 1750), p. 85.
2. Paul J. Cranefield, "The Organic Physics of 1847 and the Biophysics of Today," *Journal of the History of Medicine and Allied Sciences* 12 (1957), p. 407. See also Dennis Stillings, "California: Neither Here Nor There," *Artifex* 6:6 (1987), pp. 18–26.
3. Ivan Illich, *Medical Nemesis* (New York: Pantheon, 1976), p. 187.
4. Alastair J. Cunningham, "Mind, Body, and Immune Response," in Robert Ader, ed., *Psychoneuroimmunology* (New York: Academic Press, 1981), p. 609.
5. Cunningham, in Ader, op. cit., p. 609.

6. See "The Biodance," in Larry Dossey *Space, Time & Medicine* (Boston: New Science Library, 1982), pp. 72–81.

7. Guy Murchie, *The Seven Mysteries of Life* (Boston: Houghton Mifflin, 1978), p. 320.

8. Lincoln Barnett, *The Universe and Doctor Einstein,* revised edition (New York: Bantam, 1968), p. 39.

9. Candace B. Pert, quoted in David Kline, "The Power of the Placebo," *Hippocrates,* May/June 1988, p. 26.

10. Candace B. Pert, "The Wisdom of the Receptors: Neuropeptides, the Emotions, and Bodymind," *Advances* 3:3 (1986), pp. 8–16.

11. Lawrence LeShan, *The Dilemma of Psychology* (New York: Dutton, 1990), p. 73. Originally cited by J. McK. Cattell, presidential address to the American Psychological Association, 1895.

12. Graves, along with many of his famous contemporaries, seemed larger than life. After he obtained his medical degree in 1818, he took a continental tour, as was then the thing to do. It almost proved his undoing. In Austria he was arrested as a German spy, because his fluency in several languages made him suspect. Other adventures followed and added to his reputation. Once, while Graves was on a ship in the Mediterranean, a storm and a mutiny both arose. Graves not only quelled the mutiny, he assumed command of the ship, saving it from disaster. He was a leader and reformer in medicine all his life. He insisted on more humane treatment of hospital patients, as well as hands-on care of patients by medical students. He was iconoclastic to the end. At a time when the custom was to withhold food from febrile patients, he requested that his epitaph be, "He fed fevers." See F. H. Garrison, *History of Medicine,* 4th ed. (Philadelphia: W. B. Saunders, 1928), p. 419.

13. Garrison, op. cit., p. 420.

14. Ibid.

15. Ibid., pp. 414, 619–620, 757.

16. G. F. Hayden, "What's in a Name? 'Mechanical' Diagnosis in Clinical Medicine," *Postgraduate Medicine* 75:1 (1984), pp. 227–232.

17. Murchie, op. cit., p. 319.

18. Daniel A. Sadoff, "Value of the Human Body," letter to the editor, *New England Journal of Medicine* 308:25 (1983), p. 1543.

19. George K. Pratt, *Your Mind and You* (New York: Funk and Wagnalls, 1924), p. 1.

20. Lennart Nilsson, *The Body Victorious* (New York: Delacorte, 1987).

21. J. Silberner, "Metaphor in Immunology," *Science News* 130 (October 18, 1986), p. 254.

22. See Howard F. Stein, "The Influence of Countertransference on Decision Making and the Clinical Relationship," *Continuing Education for the Family Physician* 18:7 (1983), pp. 625–630.

23. Martha Bayles, quoted in Dennis Stillings, editorial, *Artifex* 8:1 (1989), p. 35.

24. Niels Bohr, quoted in J. A. Wheeler, "Not Consciousness but the Distinction between the Probe and the Probed as Central to the Elemental

Quantum Act of Observation," in R. G. Jahn, ed., *The Role of Consciousness in the Physical World* (Boulder, CO: Westview Press, 1981), p. 94.

25. Personal communication, source anonymous, 1989.

26. Lawrence LeShan, *The Dilemma of Psychology* (New York: Dutton, 1990), p. 137.

27. C. M. Rick, "The Tomato," *Scientific American* 239 (1978), pp. 76–87; S. H. Wittwer, "Tomato," in *Encyclopedia Americana* (Danbury, CT: Americana, 1978), vol. 26, pp. 832–833; Raymond Sokolov, "The Well-travelled Tomato," *Natural History,* June 1989, pp. 84–88.

28. J. S. Goodwin and J. M. Goodwin, "The Tomato Effect: Rejection of Highly Efficacious Therapies," *Journal of the American Medical Association* 251:18 (1984), pp. 2387–2390.

29. W. S. C. Copeman, *A Short History of Gout* (London: Cambridge University Press, 1964), pp. 38–47.

30. Goodwin and Goodwin, op. cit., p. 2388.

31. Ibid., p. 2389.

32. C. D. Jenkins, "Psychological and Social Precursors of Coronary Disease," *New England Journal of Medicine* 284 (1971), pp. 244–255.

33. *Work in America: Report of a Special Task Force to the Secretary of Health, Education, and Welfare* (Cambridge, MA: MIT Press, 1973).

34. Meyer Friedman et al., "Feasibility of Altering Type A Behavior Pattern after Myocardial Infarction," *Circulation* 66:1 (1982), pp. 83–92; Dean Ornish et al., "Effects of Stress Management Training and Dietary Changes in Treating Ischemic Heart Disease," *Journal of the American Medical Association* 249:1 (1983), pp. 54–59.

35. D. Spiegel, J. Bloom, H. Kraemer, and E. Gotheil, "Effects of Psychosocial Treatment on Survival of Patients with Metastatic Breast Cancer," *Lancet* (October 15, 1989).

36. "Unproven Methods of Cancer Management," *CA-A Cancer Journal for Clinicians* 32:1 (1982), pp. 58–61.

37. See David Cameron Duffy, "Land of Milk and Poison," *Natural History,* July 1990, pp. 4–8.

38. P. Mounsey, "Prodromal Symptoms in Myocardial Infarction," *British Heart Journal* 13 (1951), p. 215.

39. Peter F. Cohn and Eugene Braunwald, "Chronic Coronary Artery Disease," in Eugene Braunwald, ed., *Heart Disease* (Philadelphia: W. B. Saunders, 1980), p. 1410.

13. THE BODY AS MUSIC

1. Gregory of Nyssa, quoted in Paulos Mar Gregorios, *Cosmic Man: The Divine Presence; The Theology of St. Gregory of Nyssa* (New York: Paragon, 1988), p. 13.

2. Lynn Keegan, "Environment: Protecting our Personal and Planetary Home," in B. M. Dossey, L. Keegan, C. E. Guzzetta, and L. G. Kolkmeier,

Holistic Nursing: A Handbook for Practice (Rockville, MD: Aspen, 1988), pp. 183–185.

3. Mary Smith, "Human-Environment Process: A Test of Rogers' Principle of Integrality," *Advances in Nursing Science* 9:1 (1986), pp. 21–28.

4. Larry Ephron's comment provided by Brad Lemley, personal communication, September 1987.

5. Bernard Lown et al., "Basis for Recurring Ventricular Fibrillation in the Absence of Coronary Artery Disease and Its Management," *New England Journal of Medicine* 294:12 (1976), pp. 623–629.

6. The research documenting the healthful benefits of Transcendental Meditation is extensive and impressive. Further information can be obtained by writing the Department of Physiology, Maharishi International University, Fairfield, Iowa.

7. M. Cooper and M. Aygen, "Effects of Meditation on Blood Cholesterol and Blood Pressure," *Journal of the Israel Medical Association* 95:1 (1978).

8. Heinrich Heine, quoted in Macdonald Critchley, "Ecstatic and Synaesthetic Experiences during Musical Perception," in Macdonald Critchley and R. A. Henson, eds., *Music and the Brain: Studies in the Neurology of Music* (London: William Heinemann Medical Books, 1977), p. 217.

9. Susumu Ohno and Midori Ohno, "The All Pervasive Principle of Repetitious Recurrence Governs Not Only Coding Sequence Construction but Also Human Endeavor in Musical Composition," *Immunogenetics* 24 (1986), pp. 71–78. See also Susumu Ohno and Marty Jabara, "Repeats of Base Oligomers (N = 3n ± 1 or 2) as Immortal Coding Sequences of the Primeval World: Construction of Coding Sequences Is Based upon the Principle of Musical Composition," *Chemica Scripta* 26B (1986), pp. 43–49.

Grateful thanks to Charles Eagle, chairman of the Department of Music Therapy, Southern Methodist University, for introducing me to the work of Dr. Susumu Ohno.

10. Professor Ohno's process is, of course, an arbitrary one. There are many musical systems in the world, each of which would yield different results if its tones were transposed onto the genetic code and if the resulting tones were harmonized and divided into the discrete notations and beats characteristic of that particular form of music. The point is that DNA and music can be related to each other, not that the music that results from this process conforms invariably to that of a particular culture.

11. Lawrence LeShan, *The Dilemma of Psychology* (New York: Dutton, 1990), p. 19.

12. Albert Einstein, quoted in Frank Wilczek and Betsy Devine, *Longing for the Harmonies* (New York: W. W. Norton, 1989).

13. Joachim-Ernst Berendt, *Nada Brahma: The World Is Sound* (Rochester, VT: Destiny Books, 1987), p. 171.

14. Macdonald Critchley, "Musicogenic Epilepsy," in Critchley and Henson, op. cit., pp. 346–347.

15. Caelius Aurelianus, quoted in R. A. Henson, "Neurological Aspects of Musical Experience," in Critchley and Henson, op. cit., p. 6.

16. Personal communication, source anonymous, September 1990.
17. Robert S. Root-Bernstein, "Sensual Education," *The Sciences* 30:5 (1990), pp. 12–14.
18. Ibid., p. 14.
19. Ibid.
20. Ibid., p. 13.
21. Joachim-Ernst Berendt, op. cit., p. 171.

PART THREE, HEALING BREAKTHROUGHS

1. C. G. Jung, quoted in Aniela Jaffé, *The Myth of Meaning: Jung and the Expansion of Consciousness,* R. F. C. Hull, trans. (New York: Penguin, 1975), p. 146.

14, THE CASE OF THE FISHSKIN BOY:
GENES AND MEMES

1. Adapted from A. A. Mason, "A Case of Congenital Ichthyosiform Erythrodermia," *British Medical Journal* 2 (1952), pp. 422–431, and Henry L. Bennett, "Behavioral Anesthesia," *Advances* 2:4 (1985), pp. 11–21.
2. Lewis Thomas, *The Medusa and the Snail* (New York: Viking, 1979), p. 81. See Blair Justice, *Who Gets Sick: Thinking and Health* (Houston: Peak Press, 1987), p. 317.
3. D. A. Collison, "Which Asthmatic Patients Should Be Treated by Hypnotherapy," *Medical Journal of Australia* 1 (1975), pp. 776–781; quoted in Justice, op. cit., p. 315.
4. Justice, op. cit., p. 318.
5. Richard Dawkins, *The Selfish Gene* (New York: Oxford University Press, 1976).
6. See "Interview: Richard Dawkins," *OMNI* 12:4 (1990), pp. 58 ff.
7. M. Cooper and M. Aygen, "Effects of Meditation on Blood Cholesterol and Blood Pressure," *Journal of the Israel Medical Association* 5:1 (1978). [This study was also published later in the United States in the *Journal of Human Stress* and the *Journal of the American Medical Association.*]
8. John Cairns, "The Origin of Mutants," *Nature* 355: 1258 (September 8, 1988), pp. 142–145.
9. "Bacteria Show Evidence of Directed Evolution," *Brain/Mind Bulletin,* October 1988, pp. 1–2.

15, THE POWER OF BELIEF:
PSYCHIC HEALING AND THE HARVARD HEALTH SERVICE

1. Jonas Salk, quoted in Brendan O'Regan, "Healing: Synergies of Mind/Body/Spirit," *Institute of Noetic Sciences Newsletter* 14:1 (1986), p. 9.
2. Adapted from S. E. Locke and D. Colligan, *The Healer Within: The New Medicine of Mind and Body* (New York: E. P. Dutton, 1968), pp. 1–2.

3. Personal communication, Myrin Borysenko, 1991. Used with permission.

4. H. Rehder, "Wunderheilungen: Ein Experiment," *Hippokrates* 26 (1955), pp. 577–580.

5. Lawrence LeShan, *From Newton to ESP* (Wellingborough, Northamptonshire, England: Turnstone Press, 1984), pp. 173–174.

6. Adapted from Helen C. Erikson, Evelyn M. Tomlin, and Mary Ann P. Swain, *Modeling and Role-Modeling: A Theory and Paradigm for Nursing* (Englewood Cliffs, NJ: Prentice-Hall, 1983), pp. 76–77.

7. Adapted from William Mainord, Barry Rath, and Frank Barnett, "Anesthesia and Suggestion," presented at the annual meeting of the American Psychological Association, August 1983; reported in Daniel Goleman, *Vital Lies, Simple Truths: The Psychology of Self-Deception* (New York: Simon & Schuster, 1985), pp. 89–90.

8. Adapted from Henry Bennett, Hamilton Davis, and Jeffrey Giannini, "Posthypnotic Suggestions during General Anesthesia and Subsequent Dissociated Behavior," paper presented to the Society for Clinical and Experimental Hypnosis, October 1981; reported in Goleman, op. cit., p. 90.

9. Sir William Osler, quoted in Kurt Kroenke, "Polypharmacy: Causes, Consequences, and Cure," *American Journal of Medicine* 79:2 (1985), pp. 149–152.

10. Locke and Colligan, op. cit., p. 114.

11. Adapted from Wray Herbert, "Drug Death More Common in Uncommon Places," *Science News,* April 24, 1982, p. 279.

12. The concept of the Type A personality has undergone considerable refinement since it was originally proposed. Early studies suggested that the primary factor in the Type A complex was simply time awareness. However, the work of Dr. Redford B. Williams, Jr., of Duke University Medical Center has shown that the crucial factor may be the hostility, distrust, and anger harbored by the time-aware person. This may explain some of the inconsistencies of earlier Type A studies, and may come as comfort to healthy, goal-oriented, busy people who fear they may be "Type As." See Chris Raymond, "Distrust, Rage May Be 'Toxic Core' That Puts 'Type A' Person at Risk," *Journal of the American Medical Association* 261:6 (1989), p. 813.

13. Meyer Friedman et al., "Feasibility of Altering Type A Behavior Pattern after Myocardial Infarction," *Circulation* 66:1 (1982), pp. 83–92.

14. Dean Ornish et al., "Effects of Stress Management Training and Dietary Changes in Treating Ischemic Heart Disease," *Journal of the American Medical Association* 249:1 (1983), pp. 54–59.

16, THE HELPER'S HIGH:
HEALING THE SELF BY HELPING OTHERS

1. Allan Luks, "Helper's High," *Psychology Today,* October 1988, pp. 39–42.

2. Ibid., p. 40.

3. Jaak Panksepp, quoted in ibid.

4. Ibid., p. 41.

5. David C. McClelland, "Motivation and Immune Function in Health and Disease," paper presented at the meeting of the Society of Behavioral Medicine, New Orleans, March 1985.

6. Blair Justice, *Who Gets Sick: Thinking and Health* (Houston: Peak Press, 1987), pp. 256–257.

7. Joan Borysenko, "Healing Motives: An Interview with David C. McClelland," *Advances* 2:2 (1985), pp. 29–41.

17, HEALING AT A DISTANCE:
ERA III MEDICINE

1. Brad Lemley, personal communication, November 1990.

2. Sir Francis Chichester, *The Lonely Sea and the Sky* (New York: Paragon House, 1990).

3. Randolph C. Byrd, "Positive Therapeutic Effects of Intercessory Prayer in a Coronary Care Unit Population," *Southern Medical Journal* 81:7 (1988), pp. 826–829.

4. Details of the Spindrift experiments can be obtained by writing the organization at Post Office Box 5134, Salem, OR 97304-5134.

5. Dolores Krieger, *Foundations of Holistic Health: Nursing Practices* (Philadelphia: J. P. Lippincott, 1981); Dolores Krieger, *The Therapeutic Touch* (Englewood Cliffs, NJ: Prentice-Hall, 1979).

6. Daniel P. Wirth, *Unorthodox Healing: The Effect of Noncontact Therapeutic Touch on the Healing Rate of Full Thickness Dermal Wounds,* unpublished study, Healing Sciences International, 29 Orinda Way, Box 1888, Orinda, CA 94563.

7. Janet Quinn, "Therapeutic Touch as Energy Exchange: Testing the Theory," *Advances in Nursing Science* 6 (1984), pp. 42–49; Janet Quinn, *An Investigation of the Effects of Therapeutic Touch Done without Physical Contact on State Anxiety of Hospitalized Cardiovascular Patients,* doctoral dissertation, New York University, 1982, University Microfilm #DA8226788.

8. See "New Technologies Detect Effects of Healing Hands," *Brain/Mind Bulletin,* September 30, 1985, p. 3. See also John T. Zimmerman, "Laying-on-of-hands Healing and Therapeutic Touch: A Testable Theory," in M. L. Albertson, D. S. Ward, and K. P. Freeman, eds., *Paranormal Research* (Proceedings of the First International Conference on Paranormal Research, July 7–10, 1988, Colorado State University, Fort Collins, CO), pp. 656–672. Dr. Zimmerman may be reached at Bio-Electro-Magnetics Institute, 2490 West Moana Lane, Reno, NV.

9. D. W. Orme-Johnson, C. N. Alexander, J. L. Davies, H. M. Chandler, and W. E. Larimore, "International Peace Project in the Middle East," *Journal of Conflict Resolution* 32 (1988), pp. 776–812.

10. M. C. Dillbeck, C. Banus, C. Polanzi, and G. Landrith, "Test of a Field Model of Consciousness and Social Change: The TM and TM-Siddhi Program and Decreased Urban Crime," *Journal of Mind and Behavior* 9 (1988), pp. 457–486.

11. N. Pugh, K. G. Walton, and K. L. Kavanaugh, "Can Time Series Analysis of Serotonin Turnover Test the Theory That Consciousness Is a Field?" *Society of Neuroscience Abstracts* 14 (1988), p. 372; B. M. Rees, "Better Living Through Brain Chemistry?" letter to the editor, *Journal of the American Medical Association* 262:19 (1989), pp. 2681–2682.

12. See, for example, John S. Hagelim, "Is Consciousness the Unified Field? A Field Theorist's Perspective," *Modern Science and Vedic Science* 1 (1987), pp. 28–87.

13. Jacobo Grinberg-Zylberbaum and Julieta Ramos, "Patterns of Inter-hemispheric Correlation during Human Communication," *International Journal of Neurosciences* 36:½ (1987), pp. 41–55. See also "Silent 'Communication' Increases EEG Synchrony," *Brain/Mind Bulletin* 13:10 (1988), pp. 1 ff.

14. Jeanne Achterberg, *Imagery in Healing* (Boston: Shambhala, 1985).

15. William Braud and Marilyn Schlitz, "A Method for the Objective Study of Transpersonal Imagery," *Journal of Scientific Exploration* 3:1 (1989), pp. 43–63.

16. C. Norman Shealy and Caroline M. Myss, *The Creation of Health: Merging Traditional Medicine with Intuitive Diagnosis* (Walpole, NH: Stillpoint, 1988), pp. 73 ff.

17. Larry Dossey, *Recovering the Soul: A Scientific and Spiritual Search* (New York: Bantam, 1989).

18, THE PLACE OF EMPTINESS:
THE RETURN OF MIRACLES

1. Adapted from Gary Snyder, "The Etiquette of Freedom," *Sierra* 74:5 (1989), pp. 75 ff.

2. Will Steger, "Six across Antarctica," *National Geographic* 178:5 (1990), pp. 67–93. A full-length account of the trek can be found in Will Steger and Jon Bowermaster, *Crossing Antarctica* (New York: Alfred A. Knopf, 1991).

3. Snyder, op. cit.

4. Lewis Thomas, *The Atlanta Constitution*, May 3, 1980, pp. 1–3; quoted in Roger J. Bulger, "Narcissus, Pogo, and Lew Thomas's Wager," *Journal of American Medical Association* 245:14 (1981), pp. 1450–1454.

5. Lawrence LeShan, *The Medium, the Mystic, and the Physicist* (New York: Viking, 1974).

19, STANDING IN THE VOID:
PARADOXICAL AND RATIONAL HEALING

1. Paul Brunton, quoted in *Network Newsletter* no. 33 (official publication of the Scientific and Medical Network), April 1987, p. 18.

2. Saint Peter Canisius, quoted in *Parabola* 12:2, p. 128.

3. Charles Weinstock, quoted in Gregg Levoy, "Inexplicable Recoveries from Incurable Diseases," *Longevity*, October 1989, pp. 37–42.

4. Adapted from Levoy, op. cit.

5. Ibid., p. 42.

6. Funk & Wagnall's *Standard Desk Dictionary* (New York: Lippincott & Crowell, 1983), p. 474.

7. Nicholas Falletta, *The Paradoxicon* (New York: John Wiley, 1990).

8. R. D. Laing, *The Divided Self* (New York: Pantheon, 1962).

9. Adapted from St. John Dowling, "Lourdes Cures and the Medical Assessment," *Journal of the Royal Society of Medicine* 77 (August 1984), pp. 634–638.

10. Marvin R. O'Connell, "The Roman Catholic Tradition since 1545," in R. L. Numbers and D. W. Amundsen, eds., *Caring and Curing: Health and Medicine in the Western Religious Traditions* (New York: Macmillan, 1986), p. 133.

11. Kyriacos C. Markides, *The Magus of Strovolos* (New York: Arkana, 1985), p. 134.

12. Henri Matisse, quoted in Norman Cousins, "Can Creativity Heal?" *Advances* 2:3 (1985), pp. 69–72.

13. C. G. Jung, quoted in Laurens van der Post, *Jung and the Story of Our Time* (New York: Vintage, 1977), pp. 76–77.

14. Ibid., p. 30.

15. Gregory Bateson, quoted in Daniel Goleman, *Vital Lies, Simple Truths: The Psychology of Self-Deception* (New York: Simon & Schuster, 1985), p. 245.

16. Renée Weber, "Philosophical Foundations and Frameworks for Healing," *ReVision* 2:2 (1979), pp. 66–77. See also Renée Weber, *Dialogues with Scientists and Sages* (New York: Routledge & Kegan Paul, 1986).

17. See Brendan O'Regan, "Healing, Remission and Miracle Cures," Special Report of the Institute of Noetic Sciences, Sausalito, CA, May 1987.

20, THE SECRET HELPER:
THE INVISIBLE POWER WITHIN

1. Adam Fisher, "Growing Older," in Sy Safransky, ed., *A Bell Ringing in the Empty Sky: The Best of the Sun,* vol. II (San Diego: Mho and Mho Works, 1987), p. 366.

2. Aldous Huxley, *Tomorrow and Tomorrow and Tomorrow* (New York: New American Library, 1964), p. 54.

3. Thomas P. Hackett et al., "The Coronary Care Unit: An Appraisal of Its Psychological Hazards," *New England Journal of Medicine* 279 (1968), p. 1365.

4. Thomas P. Hackett and Jerrold F. Rosenbaum, "Emotion, Psychiatric Disorders, and the Heart," in Eugene Braunwald, ed., *Heart Disease: A Textbook of Cardiovascular Medicine* (Philadelphia: W. B. Saunders, 1980), pp. 1923–1943.

5. Keith W. Pettingale et al., "The Biological Correlates of Psychological Responses to Cancer," *Journal of Psychosomatic Research* 25 (1981), pp. 453–458.

6. Shelley E. Taylor, "Adjustment to Threatening Events: A Theory of Cognitive Adaptation," *American Psychologist,* November 1983, pp. 1161–1173.

7. Nick Jordan, "When to Lie to Yourself," *Psychology Today,* June 1989, p. 24 ff.

8. Elizabeth Rose Campbell, "Patricia Sun," in Sy Safransky, *A Bell Ringing in the Empty Sky: The Best of the Sun,* vol.1 (San Diego: Mho and Mho Works, 1985), pp. 278–279.

9. Hermann Hesse, *Siddhartha* (New York: New Directions, 1957), pp. 137–138.

10. Erwin Schrödinger, *My View of the World* (Woodbridge, CT: Ox Bow, 1983), p. 22.

21, THE HOSPITAL EXPERIENCE:
HOW TO BE A SURVIVOR

1. Adapted from Helen C. Erickson, Evelyn M. Tomlin, and Mary Ann P. Swain, *Modeling and Role-Modeling* (Englewood Cliffs, NJ: Prentice-Hall, 1983), p. 76.

2. Ibid.

3. Quoted in "Planetree: The New Industry Standard for Satisfying Customers," *Hospital Entrepreneurs' Newsletter* 4:2 (1988).

4. Roger S. Ulrich, "View through a Window May Influence Recovery from Surgery," *Science* 224 (1984), pp. 420–421.

5. Cathie E. Guzzetta, "Effects of Relaxation and Music Therapy on Patients in a Coronary Care Unit with Presumptive Acute Myocardial Infarction," *Heart and Lung* 18:6, pp. 609–616.

6. Henry L. Bennett, "Behavioral Anesthesia," *Advances* 2:4 (1985), pp. 11–21.

7. Ibid., p. 20.

8. S. J. Whitcher and J. D. Fisher, "Multidimensional Reaction to Therapeutic Touch in a Hospital Setting," *Journal of Personality and Social Psychology* 37:1 (1979), pp. 87–96.

9. L. D. Egbert et al., "Reduction of Postoperative Pain by Encouragement and Instruction of Patients," *Advances* 2:4 (1985), pp. 53–56; originally published in the *New England Journal of Medicine* 278 (1964), pp. 825–827.

10. See Gerard V. Sunnen, "Medical Hypnosis in the Hospital," *Advances* 5:2, pp. 5–12; see also Gerard V. Sunnen, "Miscellaneous Medical Applications of Hypnosis," in B. DeBetz and G. Sunnen, eds., *A Primer of Clinical Hypnosis* (Boston: PSG Publishing, 1985), pp. 221–226. Health care professionals will find of benefit E. Rossi and D. Cheek, *Mind-Body Therapy: Ideodynamic Healing in Hypnosis* (New York: W. W. Norton, 1988). Persons favoring a Jungian approach to hypnosis may consult an excellent book by James A. Hall, *Hypnosis: A Jungian Perspective* (New York: Guilford Press, 1989).

11. Address: Institute for the Advancement of Health, 423 Washington Street, San Francisco, CA 94111.

22, PICTURES IN THE MIND:
USING THE IMAGINATION FOR HEALING

1. For a full description of the biofeedback process and the use of handwarming techniques in treating Raynaud's disease, see Kenneth R. Gaarder and Penelope S. Montgomery, *Clinical Biofeedback* (Baltimore: Williams & Wilkins, 1977), pp. 137–142.

2. Case is from author's practice, 1986.

3. Personal communication from Charles Johnson; also quoted in *Bridgings,* his book in progress.

AFTERWORD

1. Oliver Wendell Holmes, *Medical Essays* (Boston: Houghton Mifflin Co., 1883), pp. 378–379; quoted in Fielding H. Garrison, *History of Medicine* (Philadelphia: W. B. Saunders, 1929), pp. 45–46.

2. Rainer Maria Rilke, *Letters to a Young Poet,* M. D. Herter Norton, trans. (New York: W. W. Norton, 1954), pp. 69–70.

Index

Circadian rhythm, 64–65
Cirolli, Delizia (Lourdes healing), 206–7
Cleveland Clinic, 78
Closeness, biological need for, 92–93, 96
Cogwheel rigidity, 114
Colchicine, 129–30
Computers
  as metaphor, 119, 124–26, 127–28
  in medicine, 18
  as mind, 123–24
  music program, 145–46
Congenital ichthyosis, 102, 151–52, 220
Control, 67–68, 72, 85, 86, 239–41. *See also* Biofeedback.
Coolidge, J. C., 54
Copeman, W. S. C., 129
Copenhagen Conference, 143
Coping failure, 56
Coronary artery disease, 131, 169
  bypass surgery, 15, 131
Corrigan's hammer, 112
Corrigan, Sir Dominic John, 112, 118, 123
Corvisart, Jean-Nicholas, 115, 116
Cousins, Norman, 57
CPR, 34
Crawford, Dr., 135
Creation of Health, The: Merging Traditional Medicine with Intuitive Diagnosis (Shealy & Myss), 187
Creativity, 47
Critchley, Macdonald, 144
Culture, American, 122, 213
Cunningham, Alastair J., 106
Curandera, 2

Dachau, 43
Damgaard, Jacqueline, 47
Danville, IN, 133
Davies, Paul, 13
Davis, Wade, 164–65
Dawkins, Richard, 153–54
Death

anniversary deaths, 58
bereavement and, 20, 90–91
circadian rhythm and, 64–65
education and, 69–73
elderly and "self-responsibility," 61
fear and, 78, 228
forced retirement and, 60
from emotional shock, 14, 20, 51–54
from grief, 88–96
from happiness, 53
healing and, 209–12
illicit sex and, 36–38
from meaning, 14
naturalness of, 209–13
loners and, 71–72
"no meaning" syndromes" and, 10, 11
physicians' words and, 76–77, 79, 227
social isolation and, 70–73
stages, 121
sudden, 9, 54–56, 64–65, 85, 168
twin case history, 94–95
See also Voodoo.
Defibrillator, 256
Deikman, Arthur J., 11
Demian (Hesse), 141
Democritus, 107, 145
Denial, 19, 220–22, 224
De Niro, Robert, 69
Dent, Walter, 216–18
Despair, 47, 48–56, 72, 86, 87, 90, 93
De Vaca, Alva Núñez Cabeza, 194–95, 196, 197, 199
Diagnosis, 18, 111–12
  devices, 146–47
  distant (intuitive), 187–88, 191, 192, 206
  snap, 115–16
Dickinson, Emily, 211
Dilemma of Psychology, The (LeShan), 127–28
Dillard, Annie, 194
Dimsdale, Joel E., 54–56

About the Author

Dr. Larry Dossey is a former practitioner of internal medicine with the Dallas Diagnostic Association. After graduating with high honors from the University of Texas at Austin, he received his M.D. degree from Southwestern Medical School (Dallas) in 1967. Following internship he served as a batallion surgeon in Vietnam, later completing his residency in internal medicine at the Veterans Administration Hospital and Parkland Hospital in Dallas.

Dossey was a principal organizer of the Dallas Diagnostic Association, which currently is the largest group of internal medicine practitioners in the city. He is former president of the Isthmus Institute of Dallas, an organization dedicated to exploring the convergences of science and religious thought. He is a Fellow of the Dallas Institute of Humanities and Culture, and former Chief of Staff of Medical City Dallas Hospital.

Dossey lectures widely in the United States and abroad. In 1988 he delivered the annual Mahatma Gandhi Memorial Lecture in New Delhi, India, the only physician ever invited to do so.

Dossey has published numerous articles and is the author of *Space, Time & Medicine, Beyond Illness,* and *Recovering the Soul,* which have been translated into several languages. The overall concern of these books is the interface of the human mind with health and illness. Dossey's goal has been to anchor the so-called holistic health movement in a model that is scientifically respectable and which, at the same time, answers to man's inner spiritual needs.

Dr. Dossey lives in Santa Fe with his wife Barbara, who is a nurse-consultant and the author of several award-winning books.

CREDITS

Goldstein, and A. J. Moss, *Archives of Internal Medicine,* 129:725–731, 1972. Courtesy of the Archives of Internal Medicine.

Adaptation of "Feasibility of altering type A behavior pattern after myocardial infarction" by M. Friedman, et al., *Circulation 66,* 1:83–92, 1982, reprinted by permission of the American Heart Association, Inc.

Adaptation of "Effects of stress management training and dietary changes in treating ischemic heart disease" by D. Ornish, et al., *Journal of the American Medical Association,* 249:1, 54–59, 1983. Courtesy of the *Journal of the American Medical Association.*

Adaptation of "Unexpected death in a patient who wished to die" by J. C. Coolidge, *Journal of the American Psychoanalytical Association,* 17:413–420, 1969. Courtesy of the *Journal of the American Psychoanalytical Association.*

Adaptation of "Sudden and rapid death during psychological stress: Folklore or folk wisdom?" by G. L. Engel, *Annals of Internal Medicine,* 74:771–782, 1971. Reproduced with permission.